Vaccine-nation

Poisoning the Population,
One Shot at a Time

Andreas Moritz

Other books and products
by Andreas Moritz

. . .

The Amazing Liver and Gallbladder Flush

Timeless Secrets of Health and Rejuvenation

Cancer Is Not a Disease

Lifting the Veil of Duality

It's Time to Come Alive

Feel Great, Lose Weight

Heal Yourself with Sunlight

Simple Steps to Total Health

Heart Disease No More!

Diabetes—No More!

Ending the AIDS Myth

Hear the Whispers, Live Your Dream

Sacred Santémony

Ener-Chi Ionized Stones

Ener-Chi Art

All of the above are available at www.ener-chi.com, www.amazon.com, and
other online or physical bookstores.

Vaccine-nation

Andreas Moritz

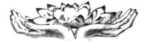

Your Health is in Your Hands

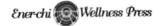

Ener-chi Wellness Press

For Reasons of Legality

The author of this book, Andreas Moritz, does not advocate the use of any particular form of healthcare but believes that the facts, figures, and knowledge presented herein should be available to every person concerned with improving his or her state of health. Although the author has attempted to give a profound understanding of the topics discussed and to ensure accuracy and completeness of any information that originates from any other source than his own, he and the publisher assume no responsibility for errors, inaccuracies, omissions, or any inconsistency herein. Any slights of people or organizations are unintentional. This book is not intended to replace the advice and treatment of a physician who specializes in the treatment of diseases. Any use of the information set forth herein is entirely at the reader's discretion. The author and publisher are not responsible for any adverse effects or consequences resulting from the use of any of the preparations or procedures described in this book. The statements made herein are for educational and theoretical purposes only and are mainly based upon Andreas Moritz's own opinion and theories. The reader should always consult with a healthcare practitioner before taking any dietary, nutritional, herbal or homeopathic supplement, or beginning or stopping any therapy. The author is not intending to provide any medical advice, nor offer a substitute thereof, and makes no warranty, expressed or implied, with respect to any product, device or therapy, whatsoever. Except as otherwise noted, no statement in this book has been reviewed or approved by the United States Food & Drug Administration or the Federal Trade Commission. Readers should use their own judgment or consult a holistic medical expert or their personal physicians for specific applications to their individual problems.

ISBN: 978-0-9845954-2-6

Published by Ener-Chi Wellness Press - Ener-chi.com, U.S.A. (Feb 2011)
Cover design by Writerforce, India (www.writerforce.com)

TABLE of CONTENTS

INTRODUCTION

I was never vaccinated against any disease. My mother, whose family included well respected medical physicians, refused to give in to the pressure of school officials and mainstream doctors who told her in no uncertain terms that she placed my brother and me in harm's way by not subjecting us to the recommended inoculations. However, her strong maternal instinct prevailed; she believed only in natural ways of developing resistance to disease.

When we eventually did experience some of the typical childhood illnesses, she told us that this was a necessary part of developing natural immunity, and we had no reason to believe otherwise. Neither my brother nor I have ever suffered from an infectious disease in over five decades, except for coming down with an occasional cold.

In the early 1980s, I began researching the theory behind the presumed need for individual and mass vaccinations and uncovered serious flaws, non-truths, and outright deceptions in the 'science' supporting it. Accordingly, I found no scientific merit at all to uphold the idea that vaccines somehow protect us against disease by stimulating the production of antibodies.

Furthermore, I learned that the data which led to the unilateral acceptance of vaccination as the only way to control infectious disease was fixed or misrepresented. Falsified evidence has given nearly everyone the impression that vaccines have prevented disease epidemics. Nothing could be further from the truth.

Take, for example, the case of the flu vaccine, which is being pushed on babies, adults and the elderly year in, year out. The *Cochrane Collaboration* regularly reviews the scientific literature comprising new studies on the effectiveness of flu vaccines. Yet, after having investigated hundreds of these studies so far, there is still no shred of evidence that the flu vaccine has protective effects compared to placebo.

The complete lack of clinical evidence to support vaccination as a method of disease prevention speaks for itself. Vaccination has not only failed to prevent disease; it has become one of its greatest contributors.

What you are about to read in this book may come as a shock to you, but please be assured that almost every statement in this book is backed by verifiable scientific facts.

Here are a few simple truths medical science and pharmaceutical companies would rather you did *not* know:

Vaccines, not viruses, cause disease

Viruses induce healing; they are not our enemies but are on our side

The 2009 swine flu outbreak is a genetically-engineered, man-made virus

AIDS was introduced to Africa so that the West could reap huge economic profits from that continent's abundant natural resources

Many vaccines are genetically engineered to actually cause disease so that 'preventive cures' can then be invented to save vast populations from these 'killer diseases'

The 'scientific truth' – that germs cause disease – and on which modern health care policies are based, is nothing but a myth

Vaccines have crippling side effects which include autoimmune disorders, sudden infant death syndrome and autism

Real scientific truth is not palatable to the pharmaceutical industry and policy makers, who are extremely intelligent people. This is no myth! But profiteering is the preserve of the canny and the cornerstone of Big Pharma, whose billions depend on perpetuating the disease myth. In other words, it reaps rich rewards for the vaccine-makers and the governments they collude with to keep us sick or to have us live in fear of falling ill.

Among the many misconceptions they have thus embedded into our collective consciousness is that vaccines are a prerequisite for good health. They have therefore made generation upon generation believe that they are life-savers that bring longevity. In this book, we shall explore the vaccination myth that has been brilliantly wielded by drug companies, who have for more than a century profited from our ignorance, fear and vulnerability.

True Lies

Vaccination is, in fact, one of the first rites of passage the human baby is subjected to – a type of 'health insurance' for the rest of our lives. In the chapters that follow, I shall explain why vaccines are, in fact, silent killers, or at the very least, disease-causing agents we could well do without.

Here are five basic myths about vaccines that will show you just how we have been collectively hoodwinked.

Myth # 1: Vaccines Prevent Disease

Truth: History presents many examples of how vaccines have caused and spread the very disease they are meant to prevent. Vaccine literature is replete with examples of individuals and groups of people who have been vaccinated against an infectious disease and have contracted the infection at a later stage.

Myth # 2: Vaccines Eradicate Disease

Truth: Infectious diseases were on the decline for months and years prior to mass immunization campaigns. Improved sanitation, hygiene and nutrition made people healthier, which also made them more naturally resistant to infections and disease. Conversely, there are numerous instances where diseases such as whooping cough and measles, believed to have been 'wiped out', have returned with a vengeance, sometimes, as in many African nations, causing epidemics despite (or because of) mass immunization campaigns.

Myth # 3: Vaccines Boost Immunity

Truth: It is unequivocal: vaccines damage the immune system. Due to their synthetic, chemical and genetic ingredients, they cause toxic overload. They weaken the immune system and actually compromise its ability to fend off disease and heal the body. Vaccines trick the immune system and induce artificial immunity. This is very different from the way natural immunity works. Tampering with this delicate process comes at a heavy price.

Myth # 4: Vaccines Are Safe

Truth: Doctors report thousands of serious vaccine reactions every year including hundreds of deaths and permanent disabilities. Long-term damage includes neurological disorders and autoimmune diseases. In fact, researchers attribute dozens of chronic immunological and neurological conditions to mass immunization programs across the globe.

Myth # 5: Vaccine Theory Is Based on Sound Scientific Principles

Truth: Louis Pasteur's Germ Theory of disease – which he retracted before his death – became the foundation of conventional medicine and vaccination. However, dozens of books written by doctors, researchers and independent investigators have revealed serious flaws in immunization theory and practice.

Just so that we don't play into the hands of profiteers and to safeguard our health, it is important to be well-informed and forearmed with knowledge of how the human body works. It is simple and does not require any scientific grounding. Often, the simple truth is begging to be understood but we would rather believe that our medical saviors come in white coats.

If that is a bitter pill to swallow, it is important to understand the motives behind the 'scientific truths' passed on from generation to generation while our children are being injected with genetically engineered biological and chemical material masquerading as vaccines.

Perhaps we are to blame as well, for don't we all have a penchant for quick-fix solutions? Taking advantage of this, vaccine science thrives on a subtle but basic fallacy. They have based their approach on bringing about lifelong immunity to an infectious-inflammatory illness without having to experience the illness first.

Their assumption is that by having antibodies in the blood for certain illness-causing germs, you are automatically protected against them. However, research has not been able to show whether protection from germs is due to the presence of antibodies or to a normal healthy immune response. It is actually much more likely that the latter is true, unless vaccine poisons have damaged or even paralyzed the immune system.

The theory that exposing the body to disease germs will trigger an immune response similar to the one generated during an actual disease experience is seriously flawed. Could nature have made such a crucial mistake as to make us dependant on injecting foreign, toxic material into our blood when we have an immune system so complex and highly developed that millions of sophisticated computers could not imitate its performance? This is rather unlikely.

Why, then, would you want to entrust your health to a cocktail of poisonous chemicals when even a somewhat weakened immune system stands a far better chance of protecting you against harm from a bout of influenza? Our body's sophisticated immune system, which has evolved over millions of years, can certainly do a better job of protecting you against disease than anything man-made. All it needs is some basic caretaking on your part. On the other hand, with each new vaccination, your immune system becomes more depleted and the side effects become more pronounced and severe. And, you may still fall ill anyway.

Pandemics Are Man-made

Before we explore this topic in detail in subsequent chapters, a brief mention about the truth behind pandemics. There is no doubt that pandemics are man-made or due to vaccination programs, starvation, poor hygiene and antibiotics, all of which compromise the immune system. Viral infection is an effect of illness, not its cause, just as bacteria are capable of infecting only unhealthy, weak or damaged cells.

Bacteria and viruses do not viciously or indiscriminately attack us. Nature does not fight against itself, if it did, we would all be dead. There is no war between humans and nature, unless of course, we try to destroy it or upset the balance of natural forces and resources and subsequently refer to the rebalancing process as disease or natural disaster. Still, the masses have fallen for this pseudo science as it has been deftly presented to them.

Analysis of the official statistics from several countries and their historical occurrences of diseases such as smallpox, diphtheria, cholera, typhoid, poliomyelitis, tuberculosis, bronchitis, tetanus, etc has revealed astounding findings. For example, diphtheria in France increased to an all-time high with the onset of compulsory immunization and immediately dropped again after the vaccine was withdrawn.

The situation was not very different in Germany when compulsory immunization for diphtheria was introduced on a mass scale between 1925 and 1944. During this period, the number of diphtheria victims increased from 40,000 to 240,000, with the incidence of infection being higher among immunized patients. In 1945, at the end of World War II, vaccines were no longer available in Germany and, within a few years, the number of cases dropped below 50,000.

Statistical data shows that most of these diseases were in rapid and continuous decline well before the introduction of immunization programs. The big epidemics began occurring when people from the rural areas moved to the big cities. The streets were used as garbage dumps, contaminating air and water and becoming the source of infectious diseases. Only a major clean-up of these congested cities and improved sanitation, hygiene and housing were able to halt the epidemics and led to drastic improvements in individual and collective health. Vaccination programs had nothing to do with it.

Big Pharma's Death Grip

So why are we led to believe that vaccines are life-savers? Spreading the notion that viruses and bacteria cause diseases is a means to keep the masses fearful and controlled. And there is big money to be made from such misconceptions.

During the 1960s, the vaccine industry was extremely under-funded because epidemics were nowhere to be found. Plans were made to manufacture new virus strains (to use them to induce cancer in animals for 'cancer research'). In truth, however, the mixing of certain viral strains, normally not occurring in nature, led to new possibilities of sabotaging the immune systems of even healthy people. The intention was to generate new illnesses and for which natural immunity is helpless. When injected into people through vaccines, these virus cocktails would shut down the immune system, destroy cell nuclei and trigger the production or human retroviruses such as HIV.

Yes, the AIDS story is one such shocking and tragic example. In 1962, UCLA scientists concocted a new virus strain to induce cancer in animals (purportedly for cancer research). They combined an animal virus with a smallpox virus that was then made into a smallpox vaccine by a major pharmaceutical company.

The vaccine was generously donated to Africa to vaccinate 125 million people. What a gesture of goodwill! Those with the weakest immune systems developed severe immune deficiency symptoms, which later were misinterpreted as AIDS diseases. Of the 125 million people who were vaccinated, 98 million developed AIDS. This new disease turned out to be huge money spinner and a bargaining chip for wealthy nations to make and keep these poor countries dependent on them by distributing condoms for population control and powerful (immune-destructive) AIDS drugs to 'cure' AIDS.

The anti-AIDS drugs that began to pour into the developing world became a means to prevent the rise and independence of the poor countries' economies. So to help these countries 'survive' the onslaught of a deadly virus and in exchange for expensive and otherwise unaffordable medications, developed countries persuaded poor countries to sign agreements to hand over important economic production rights and natural resources.

The virus myth is a convenient tool to control people. *This* is a basic truth. The only real antidote to the wily games politicians and vaccine-makers play is to educate yourself and stop playing victim in this deadly power game.

Chapter One

The Vaccine Myth

This is perhaps the most damning yet ironic testimony against vaccines, a confession that comes from none other than the man who developed the first polio vaccine – the Inactivated Poliovirus Vaccine or IPV.

Quoted in the medical journal *Science* in 1977, Dr Jonas Salk admitted before a US Senate Sub-Committee that mass inoculation against polio was the cause of most polio cases across the US since 1961.

Salk is also reported to have said that "live virus vaccines against influenza or poliomyelitis may in each instance produce the disease it intended to prevent... (and) the live virus against measles and mumps may produce such side effects as encephalitis (brain damage)."

There are many interpretations of Salk's testimony. Pro-Salk proponents point out that the scientist was referring to the "live" or oral form of the polio vaccine developed by Dr Albert Sabin in 1957 vis-à-vis his own IPV which he developed four years earlier.

However, even if that were true, it is alarming to hear from a scientist who made vaccine history that a vaccine – any vaccine – administered to vast sections of the human population could result in widespread deaths, or for that matter, any deaths at all.

We will return to this controversy in Chapter 2 on *Historical Blunders*. But for now, suffice to say that with Salk's testimony, the very premise of vaccination theory suffered a serious blow.

1. Definition of Disease

Before I illustrate how vaccines cause, and not prevent disease, let us first define 'disease' in the context of vaccines and immunity.

It has long been known that in some illnesses such as measles, chickenpox and scarlet fever, one bout of the illness usually provides lifelong immunity. A second experience with measles or scarlet fever is extremely rare.

1

Why is that so? That is because nature has gifted the human body with wonderful natural armor – an in-built immunity – that protects the body by kicking in after a bout of a particular disease.

Till modern science unraveled the secrets of the immune system, the concepts of medicine formulated in the 19th century were in part based on the understanding of medicine by the ancient Greek physician Hippocrates.

According to Hippocrates, an illness manifests itself as signs and symptoms that travel from the inner vital organs and blood circulation to the outer surface of the body. These outer symptoms manifest themselves as visible symptoms such as a rash or discharge of blood, mucus or pus.

This 'throwing off' of an illness was considered a natural healing response which returned the body to a state of balance or equilibrium. And it took place only after the inner poisons produced by the disease were cooked and digested (pepsis) during the inflammatory process.

Hippocrates's astute observations were further developed by modern science, which later uncovered the actual mechanisms of infection, inflammation and healing on these very same lines.

Disease symptoms can indeed be caused by pathogens such as bacteria and viruses. But we have also been led to think of them as enemies that we need to battle. The fact is that disease does not begin when we are exposed to or are infected with a bacterium or virus. It begins when the body begins to *respond* to a pathogen or the inflammatory-infectious process that it sets in motion. This means that disease equals healing, which is the body's way of returning to a balanced condition (homeostasis). Disease is a sure sign that the body is engaged in correcting an underlying condition that is otherwise unfavorable to its efficiency and survival.

It is critical to understand this because it turns on its head the very foundation on which vaccination theory rests. The human body's inflammatory response to disease is, in fact, a healing process. Symptoms of disease are the body's attempt to deal with accumulated toxins, waste matter, and weakened or damaged cells. The so-called pathogens appropriately assist the body in destroying and eliminating such potentially harmful materials from the system, and return the body to a healthy state of equilibrium.

Also, the magnitude of the body's response, or the severity of illness, is not only influenced by the magnitude of the resulting infection but also by the stamina of its immune system.

The healing force employed by the body is, in turn, influenced by a variety of factors such as the individual's emotional state, spiritual foundation, diet, lifestyle, environment, etc. It definitely does *not* depend on whether we have been vaccinated against infectious agents.

If the immune system is weak, the body becomes congested and toxic, or vice versa. As a result, pathogens are likely to invade the body and start the detoxification process (disease), although the majority of germ 'invasions' occur silently, without ever disturbing us. Think about it. The human body is exposed to a multitude of pathogens every day, some of them agents of (presumed) deadly diseases. If germ invasion were synonymous with disease and death, most human beings would not survive very long.

Germ Theory: Yet it is precisely this assumption on which the 19th century French scientist, Louis Pasteur, postulated this famous Germ Theory, which has since become the cornerstone of modern medicine and vaccination.

Pasteur was the first researcher to suggest that diseases are caused by germs. According to him, germs or pathogens are 'after us' because they need to prey on us for their own survival. He initially believed that infectious/inflammatory diseases are a direct result of germs feasting on us but then retracted that theory at the time of his death.

In microscopic studies of host tissues in such diseases, Pasteur, Robert Koch and their colleagues repeatedly observed that germs proliferated while many host cells were dying. These researchers concluded that germs attack and destroy healthy cells and thereby start a disease process in the body.

Although Pasteur's assumption turned out to be wrong, it had already worked its way into the world of science and got under the skin of researchers and doctors, and thus the myth that 'germs cause infection and disease' became an undisputed reality. Today, this idea continues to prevail as a fundamental 'scientific truth' in the modern medical system.

Pasteur could have just as easily concluded that bacteria are naturally attracted to sites of increased cell death, just like they are attracted to decaying organic matter elsewhere in nature.

Flies, ants, crows, vultures and, of course, bacteria are drawn towards death. This is an undisputed law of nature. Why would this be different in the body? Weak, damaged or dead cells in the human

3

body are just as prone to germ infection as an overripe or bruised fruit.

Pasteur and all the researchers that followed in his footsteps chose to think of germs either as predators or scavengers. Had they assumed that cells die for non-apparent biochemical reasons (such as toxicity buildup), our current thinking about illness and health would be quite different.

Pasteur's 'germs-are-equal-to-disease' theory basically ignored, or at least bypassed, the immune system and its awesome, if not sometimes mysterious, powers of healing.

Why it is flawed: The fact is that inflammatory/infectious illnesses cannot be attributed to germs but are located in the various human frailties that necessitate the forces of decay and death.

It is a question of subtle emphasis. While germs are indeed involved in the disease process, they are definitely not, as Pasteur assumed, intent on harming us; nor are they the actual causal agents of infectious diseases.

Germs only become aggressive to us when confronted with the poisons we create. Our body does not battle germs because they are the enemy. Likewise, germs don't wage battles against our body. In fact, there are at least 10 times as many bacteria as human cells in the body, and none of them are causing us any harm. An estimated 500 to 1000 species of bacteria live in the human gut and a roughly similar number on the skin.

As reported in the Annual Review of Microbiology, the human flora is the assemblage of microorganisms, benign and otherwise, that reside on the surface and in deep layers of skin, in the saliva and oral mucosa, in the conjunctiva, and in the gastrointestinal tracts. They include bacteria, fungi, and archaea (single-cell). The relationship between germs and humans is not merely commensal (a non-harmful coexistence), but rather is a mutualistic relationship. The microorganisms perform a host of useful functions such as fermenting unused energy substrates, training the immune system, preventing growth of parasitic species, regulating the development of the gut, producing vitamins for the host (such as biotin and vitamin K), and producing hormones to direct the host to store fats. We need them and they need us.

If the body becomes overtaxed with toxins and trapped metabolic waste products, cells may suffer severe oxygen and nutrient deprivation and subsequently become damaged or die. An immune reaction such as high fever or depletion of energy is meant to cleanse the body of these harmful substances that otherwise could lead to the eventual demise of the entire body. The presence and activity of destructive microorganisms (infection) in this situation, encouraging the inflammatory response of the body, is not only natural but desirable.

Microorganisms become only 'pathogenic' as the health of the body's organism deteriorates. Disease is built by unhealthy conditions such as buildup of toxins and waste matter, and in most cases, the disease itself becomes the medicine to cleanse the affected organs and systems of the body and return it to health.

In situations of extreme toxicity, severe physical congestion, or overuse of medical drugs and vaccines, the immune system may be so overwhelmed by the toxins it tries to eliminate that it may not be able to save the individual. In the worst-case scenario, the immune system doesn't respond to the poisons and germs at all, and no acute disease symptoms appear (fever, inflammations, pain, or other signs of infection). These individuals cannot even develop a cold or get the flu, which otherwise could serve as a relief outlet for these toxins. The result then is a chronic, debilitating illness such as congestive heart failure, lupus, arthritis or other so-called autoimmune disorders, or death.

2. The Truth About Viruses

Contrary to what conventional medicine would have you believe, viruses don't kill people. If someone is sick and also has a virus in their system, he or she is not sick because of the virus. Sickness must exist before a virus can show up.

Viruses are designed to induce healing, not illness. Symptoms such those produced by the body's effort to heal (fever, headache, dizziness, fatigue, etc), do not constitute the disease. Increasing body temperature (fever), for example, is one of the body's best methods to increase the production of immune cells to deal with toxins and then dispose of bacteria, viruses and fungi when they are no longer needed.

Influenza, for example, is the final stage of healing an underlying disease; the disease consists of a buildup of toxins, medical drugs, heavy metals, acidic waste products, dead cell material and other noxious substances that could otherwise lead to a life-threatening condition.

An infection is merely used to break down harmful substances, like metals, drugs, chemicals, pesticides, food additives and trans fatty acids from restaurant foods or readymade foods, artificial sweeteners, etc.

Usually, some of these toxic substances are broken down by the body but most of them require bacteria to dispose of them. Some other chemical compounds, however, require solvents to dissolve and remove them.

That is when the body makes viruses or allows them to be made and spread through the body via the blood and lymph. Hence, we don't need to destroy viruses; they are on our side.

Viruses are inert proteins that the body produces in order to attack and dissolve such noxious substances. Unlike bacteria, viruses are not living organisms. They are actually microscopic strips of genetic material – DNA and RNA – housed inside a capsule. Unlike bacteria, they cannot reproduce because they have no digestive system or reproductive system.

The human body makes more of these solvents when it needs to dissolve harmful substances, and it stops making them when the danger of cellular suffocation has subsided. Viruses act effectively, just like solvents in paint cleaners, and play an important role in the detoxification process. Viruses don't stop being reproduced because the body attacks them; they diminish when the body no longer needs them.

The bottom line is that viruses can only become active and increase in number in a toxic body that cannot be cleaned up by bacteria or the body itself. Allow me to reiterate something at this crucial point: The human body only creates more viruses when there is a need to mop up drug chemicals, food preservatives, air pollutants, as well as toxic metals such as mercury and aluminum, pesticides, antibiotics and animal parts that are present in every vaccine.

To protect itself, the body may store an enormous number of different viruses but they remain inactive till a need arises for them to become active and spread to do their important work. The body removes and disposes of most of them once the detoxification process is complete. It is commonly believed that the immune system produces antibodies to combat and destroy viruses, but this may not be true. More on the true role of antibodies later.

Vaccinating an individual to invoke antibody production interferes with the body's most basic healing mechanisms, and I

6

consider it to be one of modern medicine's most dangerous weapons – truly a weapon of mass destruction.

3. Who's The Life-Saver?

In the scenario where the immune system has successfully restored the body's functions, the body is healthier and stronger than before. This bestows what many call acquired immunity but doesn't necessarily involve immunity against specific germs. It may just as well mean the body is now healthy and free of toxins, and hence there is no further need for germs to evoke the body's cleansing and healing response. Many people argue that the body has then acquired immunity to the germs that initiated the rescue mission, but, in truth, it is the heightened state of health and vitality that keeps the body from falling ill again.

Vaccine science has pursued the question of how we can bring about lifelong immunity to an infectious/inflammatory illness without having to experience the illness first.

The assumption is that by evoking production of antibodies to combat certain illness-causing germs, you are automatically protected against them. However, modern medicine has not been able to prove whether protection from the germs is due to the presence of antibodies or to a naturally healthy immune response which is primarily intended to purify and heal the congested, damaged tissues. It is actually much more likely that the latter is true, unless vaccine poisons have damaged or even paralyzed the immune system. (We shall explore the issue of immunity in Chapter 3: Is There A Conspiracy?: The War Within)

The current germ theory suggests that only when the number of germs or their rate of growth exceeds a certain threshold are they then recognized by the immune system, resulting in the formation of antibodies specific to the particular microbe. Or could there be another explanation as to why antibodies are produced?

A large presence of germs indicates that the cell tissue has become damaged or weak due to the accumulation of acid waste or another kind or injury. At that level of infection, things begin to spin seriously out of control and a tribe of germs proliferates wildly and provokes the full healing force of our immune system. This is what doctors call an 'acute inflammatory response'.

Symptoms usually include fever, release of stress hormones by the adrenal glands, increased flow of blood, lymph and mucus, and a streaming of white blood cells (lymphocytes) to the inflamed area (wound). The afflicted person feels sick and may experience pain, nausea, vomiting, diarrhea, weakness and chills.

The sweating out and throwing off of the illness is a natural response by the body that reflects a healthy immune system. In other words, the illness actually shows that the body is capable of successfully dealing with an unhealthy condition. This mandates that the illness is allowed and supported, not suppressed and aggravated. A really sick person would no longer be able to produce such healing responses.

Once we have successfully passed the challenge of a particular illness, it is less likely that we will experience it again. Somehow the illness and our response to it have made us immune to its recurrence.

It is highly doubtful that vaccination can do the same for us by forcing the body to make antibodies for some germs that appear to be causing an infection, thus protecting the individual against an infectious disease in the future.

On the contrary, it has been shown, time and again, that despite vaccination against a particular illness, the vaccinated individual may develop the very illness he is supposedly protected against. The proven fact that the mere presence of antibodies to a specific pathogen does not protect a person against infection should have raised serious doubts among medical professionals and lay people alike that the vaccine theory is seriously flawed or invalid. We cannot have it both ways; antibodies either protect us or they don't. Why do so many vaccinated people with high antibody presence for whooping cough and measles develop these diseases when vaccine science insists that these antibodies serve as protection against them? It is obvious that we are not being told the truth.

In Chapters 2 and 3 on Historical Blunders and Is There A Conspiracy?, we shall look at instances in the past where mass vaccination during or after an epidemic has in fact increased the incidence of an illness, apart from killing large swathes of the population. In many cases, these deaths have been directly linked to the introduction of a specific virus, as well as animal parts used to grow the vaccine, and toxic chemicals and metals contained in vaccines, into the human body.

4. Antibodies due to Vaccine Injury

If vaccines can cause death and paralysis in some, they can certainly cause injuries in many others, even if these harmful side effects are not immediately recognized. When tissues are injured, the body initiates a wound healing process that may involve an infection during which pathogenic germs help decompose the damaged or dead cells. Wound healing requires that the body dispatches immune cells, and yes, antibodies, to the site of injury.

Scientific research clearly demonstrates that lymphocyte participation in wound healing is a dynamic and distinctive process. The wound repair process is a very complex and highly ordered sequence of events that encompasses haemostasis, inflammatory cell infiltration, tissue regrowth and remodeling. If we want to successfully heal, we need to allow this ordered sequence to unfold without interference.

Wound healing follows tissue destruction, and antibodies bind to wounded tissues, which facilitates the engulfment of damaged tissues by macrophages, another important group of immune cells. B cells in particular, which produce and dispatch antibodies to damaged tissues, are involved in the process of wound healing. In fact, a recent study published in Immunology (2009 Nov) clearly shows that proper wound healing is impossible without the active participation of antibodies. For example, the researchers detected the antibody complex, immunoglobulin G1 (IgG1), binding to wounded tissues.

The fact that the body produces antibodies to heal damaged tissues raises a crucial point that is sufficiently convincing to challenge the current vaccine theory. What if antibodies are not at all produced to fight off germs, such as viruses or bacteria, but instead to repair the injuries caused by toxins, acidic waste matter, chemicals in foods, drugs, the poison fluoride in drinking water, etc?

In the case of vaccine shot injury, not unlike any other injury, antibodies must be produced in order to heal the tissue damage caused by injecting toxic chemicals, such as formaldehyde, anti-freeze agents, antibiotics and the deadly cocktail of preservatives they contain, directly into the blood stream. Just sticking a needle into someone's arm is already enough to evoke the body's inflammatory response which is necessary to heal the afflicted arm wound. In most cases, the body can repair the damage. However, if the immune system is weak to begin with, the vaccine injury may be fatal. A 2004 investigation has revealed that one in 500 children are born with a problem with their immune system that could cause serious or life-threatening reactions when vaccinated (Journal of Molecular Diagnostics, 2004 May, Volume 6 no 2, Pp 59-83). How many parents know whether their child has a weak immune system? Most parents and doctors are not aware of this risk because such information would seriously jeopardize the vaccine industry.

The other thing parents are not being told is that the viruses, bacteria, fungi and chemical toxins in one single vaccination force the immune system to respond and make antibodies that can cause genetic switches to be turned on and off. In the case of a developing child, this may lead to irreparable damage to the mind and/or body of that child. In the United States a child receives 36 vaccinations before age five, and one child in 91 develops autism. Eight deaths per 1000 in children below five years of age are due to vaccinations. In comparison, in Iceland a child receives 11 vaccine shots while only one child in 11,000 develops autism, and only four children per 1000 die as a result of being vaccinated. In 1980, a child received eight vaccinations and autism was rare. Today, Iceland ranks at # 1 in the world with respect to lifespan and the United States ranks at # 34. You can do the math and draw your own conclusions. More about the vaccine-autism link later.

All vaccine-makers claim that an increase in antibody production in the body results from the body's exposure to a presumed pathogen (disease-causing germ). Given the very design of the body's healing system (immune system), and supported by the aforementioned scientific research, it is just as likely that antibody production following vaccination is due to the necessity to heal the injuries caused by the toxins in the vaccine.

The question that arises is why do we refer to antibodies as being 'anti' something when the body uses them to heal itself? I propose to call them 'probodies', for they are primarily not against something, but rather for something. They are made and secreted by blood plasma cells that are derived from the B cells of the immune system to heal injury caused by a buildup of toxins. Vaccines are packed full with toxins, fragments of animal parts, and other foreign material that the body must recognize as antigens.

Antigens are usually proteins or polysaccharides. They are typically 'bound' at specific binding sites of an antibody. Antigens can consist of parts (coats, capsules, cell walls, flagella, fimbrae, and toxins) of bacteria, viruses, and other microorganisms. Non-microbial antigens can include pollen, egg-white, animal dander, plant toxins, etc.

Vaccines, which may include many different antigens, are intended to raise antibody production to raise the body's so-called 'acquired immunity'. However, as of now, there is no double blind control study to show that vaccines offer a higher level of immunity than by taking a placebo or by doing nothing at all. I wonder why there has never been such a study. The Centers for Disease Control and Prevention (CDC)'s official argument against studying the harmful effects of vaccines in humans is that any such a study (on humans) is 'unethical'.

And so I ask whether it is ethical to inject hundreds of millions of unsuspecting people, including children, each year with vaccines that have never been proven effective in preventing infectious disease, but on the contrary have been clearly shown to make them ill? Aren't we allowing double standards and legalization of mass experimentation to override this legitimate question by parents who want no harm done to their child: "Where is the proof that vaccines improve my child's immunity and keep it healthy?" Do we have to take the doctor's word for it?

Take the answer from someone who is best suited to have an objective insider's perspective. Dr. Marcia Angell disclosed after two decades as an editor for The New England Journal of Medicine: "It is simply no longer possible to believe much of the clinical research that is published, or to rely on the judgment of trusted physicians or authoritative medical guidelines."

The fact of the matter is that vaccines inhibit and systematically destroy the immune system. And there is real scientific evidence to prove it; evidence that has not been manipulated to yield more power and resources to vested interest groups.

5. Vaccines Suppress Immunity

One careful study of illness patterns observed in 82 healthy infants before and after vaccination was published in Clinical Pediatrics (1988). In this study conducted in Israel, researchers compared the incidence of acute illnesses in the 30-day period following DTaP vaccine (against Diphtheria, Tetanus, Pertussis) to the incidence in the same children for the 30-day period prior to receiving the vaccine. The three-day period immediately following vaccination was excluded because children frequently develop fever as a direct response to vaccine toxins. According the researchers, the babies experienced a dramatic increase in fever, diarrhea, and cough in the month following DTaP vaccine compared to their health before the shot.

It is relatively easy to observe whether vaccines have any negative effect on white blood cells, which form the body's primary immune system. Accordingly, a more recent peer-reviewed study, published in the New England Journal of Medicine in May 1996, revealed that tetanus vaccine produces a drop in T Cells and thus disables the immune system in HIV patients. Of course, this means, the vaccine can damage anyone's immune system, not just in those whose immune system has already been compromised. It is anyone's guess what a compromised immune system can lead up to.

In 1992, the New Zealand Immunization Awareness Society (IAS) conducted a survey study to find out how many of its members' children were suffering from health problems. Among other disease conditions of an impaired immune system, the vaccinated versus unvaccinated children suffered:

- five times more asthma
- nearly three times more allergies
- over three times more ear infections
- over four times more apnea and near miss cot death
- nearly four times more bouts of recurring tonsillitis
- ten times more hyperactivity

I can certainly vouch for these findings. In all the 37 years I have been involved with the natural health field, I have rarely seen unvaccinated children who were also autistic, hyperactive, or suffered from asthma, ear infections, allergies and tonsillitis. On the other hand, I have witnessed these occurrences among vaccinated children at alarmingly high rates.

A study published in PEDIATRICS Vol. March 1998 (pp. 383-387) found that acute encephalopathy followed by permanent brain injury or death was associated with measles vaccines. A total of 48 children, ages 10 to 49 months, met the inclusion criteria after receiving measles vaccine, alone or in combination. Eight children died, and the remainder had mental regression and retardation, chronic seizures, motor and sensory deficits, and movement disorders.

In September 2010, CNN reported that nine-month-old twins in Ghaziabad, India died within minutes of receiving a measles vaccine. Avika and Anika Sharma were given the vaccinations at a private nursing home by Dr Satyaveer Singh. Within about 15 minutes, both little girls were dead. The Indian Medical Association's local president Dr Santosh Aggrawal, who visited the hospital after the incident, confirmed that the health of the twins deteriorated after being administered the vaccine. He said, "The doctor had a fresh supply of the vaccine. Still there could be something wrong with the batch of vaccines. Similar deaths have been reported from Kanpur and Lucknow," he added. When asked for comment, investigators said: "This is a case of adverse event following immunization ... This is not a new phenomenon ..."

One problem with determining the number of vaccine injuries or vaccine-caused deaths is that only a tiny fraction of the reactions are actually made known. Studies have estimated that only between 1 and 10 percent of side effects are ever reported. Doctors and hospitals are very reluctant to blame vaccines for the sudden onset of disease or death. They still consider vaccination to be the greatest medical achievement of all times. Besides, it is not good PR to admit that the medical treatment is responsible for causing brain damage or death. Blaming accidental occurrence of disease instead of vaccines on these side effects automatically works as a waiver of liability that extends to all acts of negligence.

Accordingly, most people have no idea how serious an issue vaccine injury has become. Unsuspecting parents may be taking their perfectly healthy children to the doctor, and moments or several days later they find them to be crippled or deceased. For the medical industry, it is collateral damage or collateral gain (losing or gaining a potential patient). For a parent, it is unimaginable trauma.

If such obvious injuries and immediate death can be inflicted upon children by the measles vaccine, I ask what other more subtle and unnoticeable disease-generating conditions can it bring on that eventually lead to cancer, diabetes, heart disease, liver and kidney failure, etc years later?

Instead of filling up a child with obviously unsafe and untested vaccines and thereby risking their health and lives, we may be better off nursing them through a few typically mild and harmless childhood diseases. Doing not much at all and letting nature take its course may actually strengthen their natural immunity and improve their health in the long term.

Germs produce toxins (antigens) which trigger an inflammatory response to help heal an underlying condition that the body may not be able to heal without employing their assistance. The plasma cells produce antibodies binding to these antigens where appropriate, which facilitates healing. B cells, lymphocytes, macrophages, and antibodies are all intricately involved in this healing process, which includes the neutralization and removal of toxins. The immune system is not a war machine that is equipped with weapons to target and destroy invading enemies; on the contrary, it is a highly sophisticated healing system whose sole purpose is to return the body to a state of balance and harmony (homeostasis).

It is important to mention here that not all vaccines are useless or harmful. For example, 'homeopathic vaccines' which are made up either from things that cause the disease, or from products of the disease, such as pus, have been shown to lead to remarkable recoveries.

In fact, many people bitten by poisonous snakes are saved by administering them the venom taken from that particular species of snake. According to Wikipedia, the acquisition of human immunity against snake venom is one of the oldest forms of vaccinology known to date (about AD 60, Psylli Tribe). Even today, people of the aboriginal tribes intentionally cut their skin and expose the wound to dirt to build a strong, natural resistance to toxins present in their environment. Wild animals often follow similar self-immunization practices.

Snake venom is highly modified saliva consisting of proteins, enzymes, substances with a cytotoxic effect, neurotoxins and coagulants. When self-injected, Eastern diamondback venom develops a high IgG neutralizing antibody for several rattlesnake species. Exposure to the snake poison induces immunity against future rattlesnake bites. The immunity is caused by the body generating antiserum to neutralize the toxic effects of the snake serum. This principle applies to every toxin that the body ingests. Simply put, our body produces specific blood proteins (antibodies) to bind to and neutralize toxins and to heal the injury caused by the toxins. The achieved cellular immunity (ability to reproduce the same antidote serum in the case of another snake bite) protects the body against future exposure to the same toxin, unless the degree of exposure greatly exceeds the body's detoxification and compensation ability.

This happens especially when numerous vaccines are administered within a short time frame i.e. several months or years. As the previously mentioned research has shown, children in Iceland or Norway who only receive a total of 11 vaccines have a much lower risk of developing autism or dying than children in the US. Federal public health officials recommend that children should get a total of 69 doses of 16 vaccines from the day of their birth to age 18. We have already seen that children have a much higher incidence of asthma, allergies, ear infections, tonsillitis, and other serious ailments after they are vaccinated.

A child, who comes into the world with virtually no functional immune system, and who receives dozens of vaccine shots filled with toxic compounds, will subsequently suffer short-term damage as well as long-term damage, some of which will show up as autism, cancer, diabetes, heart disease, multiple sclerosis, Alzheimer's disease, etc years later. Perhaps, this is the reason that the United States population ranks so low with regard to life expectancy (#49) when compared with countries like Iceland, Sweden and Switzerland, where fewer vaccinations are given and where more informed parents refuse them because of the mounting evidence of widespread vaccine injuries among the population.

Is it just coincidence that the US ranks first in health care costs and spends more than twice the amount on health care as other developed nations? Why are Americans so much sicker than people from other countries, in spite of having the most advanced health care system in the world? Or is it because of that?

Barbara Loe Fisher, founder of the National Vaccine Information Center, recently described this dilemma in one sentence: "The truth is, nobody knows how many vaccine victims there are in America, how many of the 1 in 6 learning disabled children; or the 1 in 9 with asthma; or the 1 in 100 who develop autism; or the 1 in 450 who become diabetic, can trace their chronic inflammation, disease and disability back to vaccine reactions that have been dismissed by public health officials and doctors for the past century as just "a coincidence".

Planting dead or alive microbes into the blood stream in order to acquire immunity against future infections is entirely different than acquiring immunity by going through the entire course of a disease. There are no real shortcuts to immunity.

At this point, I would like to emphasize that the mere presence of specific antibodies cannot protect the human body against illness; only the cellular immune system can. And to reiterate, it accomplishes this not through the force of fighting but through the power of healing. Although science has learnt how to bestow antibodies through vaccination (by injuring the body), it mistakenly assumes it is bestowing the immune strength that can only be developed through the experience of a particular illness. Tricking the body's immune system does not work; allowing nature to take its course does.

The bottom line is that antibodies against pathogens alone are not sufficient to produce immunity. It is well-known that several diseases such as herpes outbreaks may keep recurring despite high antibody levels.

Whether or not antibodies are present, immunity to these infectious diseases can only be conferred by our cellular immune system. The theory that exposing the body to germs will trigger an immune response similar to the one generated during an actual disease experience is seriously flawed. (See Chapter 3: Is There A Conspiracy?: The War Within)

Therefore, while questioning the very premise of vaccine theory, the question we must instead ask is: Who is the real life-saver? The vaccine? Or a healthy immune system?

However, vaccine proponents almost completely bypass the role of the immune system, choosing instead to reduce it to a mechanism that produces antibodies, a robotic army of soldiers that moves in as soon as there is a 'germ invasion'. Ergo, it is the vaccines that induce immunity! Or so they would have us believe, 'they' being those who profit from other people's sickness.

They want to distract us from discovering and utilizing all the other factors responsible for bestowing a healthy, vital immune system, including vitamin D produced in response to sun exposure, exercise, good nutrition, sufficient sleep, clean water and air, choosing a more relaxing, less stressful lifestyle, etc.

Having produced antibodies to a particular substance, food, or vaccine does not ultimately determine whether an illness such as an infection or allergy will actually occur. For example, people who have multiple personality disorder may be severely allergic to orange juice (allergen) while exhibiting one personality, yet when they suddenly switch to a different personality, these very same antibodies no longer trigger an allergic reaction. They may also be diabetic in one personality, and a few minutes later, they are diabetes-free. Women may even have different menstrual cycles while passing through their different personalities.

There is another example. A normal person who is allergic to cat dander and comes into contact with the proteins of the cat hair triggers the production of antibodies and subsequent inflammatory reaction. However, as it happens frequently, this person may only be allergic to white or orange cats, but not to black cats, or vice versa.

Typically, a previous traumatic incidence involving a white cat, such as its death, may have led to the production of antibodies. Whenever the person touches a white cat, the body generates the antibody reaction based on the memory of that previous emotional trauma. And since black cats are not part of this memory, touching a black cat will not trigger an allergic reaction.

Along this line, something similar may happen to a person who suffers from an allergic reaction to gluten whenever he eats bread, but he doesn't have a problem with eating pasta that also contains gluten.

In other words, there is no way of telling for sure whether the mere presence of antibodies generated by a vaccine against the mumps or measles virus will offer any protection. The entire vaccine theory is based on the idea that the presence of such specific antibodies in the blood stream bestows immunity against these diseases. For example, the research data collected during the most recent outbreak of mumps shows without a doubt that having antibodies against such viruses has zero protective benefits without the underlying cellular immunity produced by going through the disease. Not only that. We know that 770 out of the 1,000 people sickened with mumps were fully vaccinated against it and 230 weren't. Not having any vaccine-induced antibodies against the mumps virus apparently provides a much better guarantee to remain disease–free than having them. To say it bluntly, the unvaccinated are obviously better protected than the vaccinated. The bottom line is that vaccines increase one's chances of viral infection, not decrease it.

6. Infecting Volunteers

In 2006, a team of research scientists from Duke's Center for Genomic Medicine, University of Virginia, University of Michigan and the National Center for Genomic Resources, conducted a project with a total of 57 volunteers. The participants were infected through the nose with either a cold virus, an influenza virus or a respiratory syncytial virus. Twenty-eight volunteers subsequently developed flu- or cold-like symptoms.

The aim of the study was to determine whether any of the more than 20,000 genes in the human body underwent any changes in response to the viral exposure. Accordingly, among the 28 study participants who ended up getting sick, researchers found a set of about 30 genes that were turned on in response to having been infected with a virus. In the 29 people who never developed symptoms, there were no changes to the group of genes.

I am not going to comment about the genomic implications of the study since it is well-known that foreign protein fragments (called viruses) can turn on genes. I rather want to pose the question why the 29 participants who never developed any symptoms remained healthy in spite of the same degree of exposure to the disease-causing germs. Why were the viruses in these individuals unable to turn on these same 30 genes? If an influenza virus successfully enters the body, what decides whether or not the body will meet the intrusion with a flurry of antibodies and the mounting of an inflammatory response? The answer is quite simple. Obviously, the healthy participants didn't fall sick due to the viruses because viruses cannot make healthy people sick. Their genes remained unaffected by viral intrusion.

On the other hand, why did the other group of 28 participants fall ill? The answer is that only unhealthy people can fall sick because of viruses. As mentioned before, viruses can trigger a powerful cleansing and healing response in the body that returns a congested, toxic body into a more balanced condition.

Before assuming that viruses cause disease, rather than restore a person's failing health, it would be wise to briefly examine why the so-called epidemics really occur. During the 2009 H1N1 epidemic, the media reported that several toddlers had developed swine flu symptoms and subsequently died. As it turned out, these children had never before been in contact with anyone who carried the H1N1 virus or any other infectious virus. However, these children all suffered from a serious pre-existing condition, such as heart disease.

Likewise, there are thousands of children that test positive for the HIV virus, yet both their parents test negative. Even some newborn babies test positive for HIV while their parents don't. If nobody infected these children, how did they get infected? This is an inconvenient question to ask health officials because it completely contradicts the germ theory which states that pathogenic germs are transmitted from person to person. In truth, a healthy, strong immune system and toxin-free body will not require to contract an infection to return to a balanced state, and therefore will remain unaffected by pathogens.

There are a number of reasons why children may fall ill. First, their blood never had the chance to be properly cleansed by the mother's placenta because the umbilical cord was clamped right after birth instead of 40-60 minutes later. Early clamping also causes the infant's blood oxygen to be at no more than 60 percent of normal levels.

Second, a child's evolving immune system is injured by multiple vaccines right from birth, including the unnecessary hepatitis B vaccine (given for a disease children hardly ever develop, and for which they require revaccination anyway when they are a little older because of diminished antibodies). Injecting aluminum and formaldehyde contained in this vaccine into newborn babies should worry every parent and doctor.

Third, babies who are not breastfed, or the mother is unhealthy herself and does not produce good quality breast milk, cannot build a normal healthy immune system.

Fourth, at doctor's orders, babies are kept out of the sun for at least six months after birth and therefore become vitamin D deficient. By contrast, mothers in Africa regularly take their newborn babies into the sun, and thus these infants rarely suffer from vitamin D deficiency. Vitamin D is essential for building a strong immune system. A recent study by researchers at Oregon State University showed that vitamin D is so crucial to the functioning of your immune system that vitamin D's ability to boost immune function and keep the body protected and healthy has been conserved in the genome for over 60 million years of evolution.

"The existence and importance of this part of our immune response makes it clear that humans and other primates need to maintain sufficient levels of vitamin D," said Adrian Gombart, an associate professor of biochemistry and a principal investigator with the Linus Pauling Institute at Oregon State University.

Vitamin D, which is actually a steroid hormone produced in large amounts as a result of regular sun exposure, regulates over 2,000 genes. It acts like a switch that turns the body's healing system on and keeps it active and responsive. If vitamin D becomes deficient, the switch turns off and the body's healing and detoxification ability drops significantly. This, in turn, blocks the body's ability to heal and rid itself of toxins, including those produced by micro-organisms.

As a result, a vitamin D deficient person, child or adult, will become so congested with toxins that an increasing number of cells become damaged or die, an infection therefore becomes necessary to invoke a powerful healing and cleansing response. As seen in the above mentioned examples, it doesn't matter whether the affected person has received a virus or bacterium from someone else, although this may certainly accelerate the speed with which disease symptoms occur. Our body is home to numerous species of bacteria and many viral materials that remain well hidden and dormant, but become activated and multiplied should their assistance be required. Typically, the resulting infection will come to an end once the cleansing and repair job has been accomplished.

However, in a person who is severely vitamin D deficient, the inflammation may escalate to a degree that can turn out to be fatal. Vitamin D normally prevents the 'adaptive' immune response from over-reacting and reduces inflammation. In other words, it keeps the immune system in check, and suppresses it if necessary.

Young children and elderly people who do not expose their skin to the sun enough, or who use sunscreens to block off the vitamin D-generating ultraviolet rays of the sun, are particularly susceptible to an over-reactive immune system.

The above are the first to get a winter cold or the flu. Have you ever wondered why there is no flu season in the summer? It's because most people spend more time in the outdoors during the warmer summer months which allows them to replenish their vitamin D stores and makes them less prone to falling ill.

A paper covering research conducted at major American universities has shown that many common diseases are linked with low levels of vitamin D. According to the paper which was published in the Journal of American College of Cardiology in 2008 (2008:52:1949–56), low vitamin D levels have been documented in patients with myocardial infarction, stroke, heart failure, and cardiovascular disease. Chronic vitamin D deficiency can cause secondary hyperparathyroidism, which predisposes patients to inflammation, insulin resistance, metabolic syndrome, and diabetes mellitus.

Furthermore, in the United States, cancer rates and cases of multiple sclerosis are more prevalent in the Northeast, where people tend to be more vitamin D deficient than in the South or Southwest, where it is a lot warmer and sunnier during the winter months.

Also, obese persons, smokers, and those using medications (e.g. anticonvulsants, glucocorticoids, antiretrovirals), as well as the institutionalized, are more likely to be vitamin D deficient. Persons who are dark-skinned but reside in less sunny countries or states, or who neglect spending a lot of time in the sun, are often the most vitamin D deficient. Hence their generally higher risk of infection, cancer, heart disease and diabetes.

A study published in the Virology Journal in 2008, and confirmed by another study in 2009 that involved 19,000 Americans, found that people with the lowest blood vitamin D levels reported having significantly more recent colds or cases of the flu.

In conclusion, lead author of the study, Dr Adit Ginde, stated: "The findings of our study support an important role for vitamin D in prevention of common respiratory infections such as colds and the flu. Individuals with common lung diseases, such as asthma or emphysema, may be particularly susceptible to respiratory infections from vitamin D deficiency."

Why do we need to expose our bodies to potentially life-threatening vaccines for all kinds of diseases when we can remain disease-free by exposing our skin to the sun ? (See also my book, Heal Yourself with Sunlight).

And there is more on the role of Vitamin D later.

7. What's In That Vial?

So briefly, what is this highly-potent, poisonous cocktail introduced into the human body? Injected, taken orally or even sniffed as in the case of some flu vaccines, this concoction attempts to induce immunity by forcing bits and pieces of disease-causing agents or pathogens into the body.

These are foreign bodies such as a bacteria, viruses or genetic material from these pathogens, which are usually nurtured and cultured in the bodies of infected animals, to force an immunological response.

As soon as the human body detects the presence of a foreign body (one which does not have a 'self-marker') or an antigen, it produces antibodies to neutralize these toxins, foreign cells and injurious materials, and to heal any injuries that they may have caused.

Antibodies are protein molecules that bind to antigens and may be disease-specific. As soon as the antigen and antibody lock into each other, the body's immune system is triggered to fight the intruder, according to theories taught at medical schools.

It is assumed that once an individual's bloodstream contains the antibodies (either forcibly produced by vaccines or naturally produced from a previous bout of a disease) to a particular pathogen, the human body is protected against the disease 'caused' by that particular pathogen for life.

However, there is a crucial difference in immunity acquired naturally (from a previous bout) and that which is thrust upon an unsuspecting immune system. The natural routes for pathogens to enter the body are the mucous membranes of nostrils, the mouth, the lips, the eyelids, the ears, the genital area, and the anus. Injecting pathogens directly into the blood is an unnatural route and act of violence that disrupts, and interferes with, the very design of the body's self-preserving, protective mechanisms.

These mucus membranes form the body's first line of defense to trap and digest microorganisms (using enzymes) that offer no benefit to the host as long as the cells and organs remain well nourished and healthy.

Please be reminded at this point that bacteria and viruses do no harm to the body. They become pathogenic (disease–generating) only when the body's level of toxicity has led to considerable cell damage or cell decay and an infection becomes necessary to decompose the cell debris and stimulate the immune system to repair and heal the damage. The mucus membranes form an essential part of the body's detoxification system to ensure that this doesn't need to happen.

Bypassing this first line of defense, which is also called 'IgA immune system', leaves gaping holes in the body's self-protective 'armor'. It doesn't take too well to artificial immunization measures and hence revolts in many ways. One way is by actually causing the disease the vaccine was meant to prevent.

Getting the disease for which you receive the vaccine, such as mumps, may actually be a blessing for the afflicted and bestow true immunity to the disease. This may account for some of the disease-preventing effects of vaccines that have been witnessed in a small number of vaccinated individuals. Unfortunately, the vast majority of the vaccinated population doesn't fall sick. If it did, vaccination could actually have some value. However, if an adjuvant such as aluminum or squalene is added to the vaccine, which is now typical for most vaccines, it can cause your immune system to overreact to the introduction of the organism you are being vaccinated against.

On such occasions, the human body is helpless against the foreign material and is overwhelmed by the antigens and the resulting overreaction of the immune system. This often gives rise to debilitating symptoms (among the agents most often introduced through vaccines is thimerosal, which is linked to neurological damage in the brain), crippling side effects (See Chapters 5 & 6: The Vaccine Hangover & Autism: Merury Assault) and even life-threatening conditions.

Despite documented evidence that links vaccination to disease and injury, modern medicine insists that vaccines are a type of 'health insurance'. But just so you know your facts, here is a brief look at what these chemicals contain.

Antigen: At the crux of every vaccine is the disease-causing microorganism or pathogen against which immunity is sought to be induced.

Preservatives: Preservatives are used to increase the shelf-life of a vaccine by preventing bacteria and fungi from invading it. In the US, the FDA allows the use of three preservatives: phenol, 2-phenoxyethanol and thimerosal. (See Chapter 6: Autism: Mercury Assault)

Adjuvants: Adjuvants enhance the body's immune response immediately after the vaccine is introduced. Though highly dangerous and known to even cause cytokine storms that lead to swift death, pharma companies continue to use adjuvants as 'boosters' in their vaccines.

Another compelling reason for the use of adjuvants is that these chemicals, by turbo-charging vaccines, allow drug companies to use less of the antigen in each dose so that they can make more doses. Do the math: More doses means bigger profits.

Aluminum salts are the most widely used adjuvants employed by drug manufacturers. They include: aluminum phosphate, aluminum hydroxide, aluminum hydroxyphosphate sulfate and potassium aluminum sulfate or simply alum.

Till recently, aluminum salts were the only adjuvants vaccine-makers in the US were allowed to use. However, with the FDA toying with the idea of allowing squalene as an adjuvant, there is growing alarm that this chemical, which played havoc with US Gulf War veterans, may be licensed for mass use in the US. (See Chapter 3: Is There A Conspiracy?: The War Within).

Additives or Stabilizing Agents: Stabilizing agents protect vaccines from getting damaged or losing their efficacy under certain conditions such as freeze-drying and heat. They also prevent the antigen from sticking to the side of the vaccine vial, and the components of the vaccine from separating.

Common additives include sugars such as sucrose and lactose; amino acids such as glycine, monosodium glutamate; and proteins such as gelatin or human serum albumin.

Concerns regarding these additives center around the use of gelatin, human serum albumin and material derived from bovines, especially cows. While gelatin is suspected to precipitate hypersensitivity reactions, human serum albumin (derived from dead human fetuses) could introduce pathogens into the body.

Material taken from cattle came into focus with the outbreak of Bovine Spongiform Encephalopathy or 'mad cow disease' in England in the 1980s. I've discussed this controversy in detail at the end of this chapter.

Residual Agents: Residual agents are used during the production process to inactivate the live pathogen and to culture the virus. They are eventually removed from the vaccine, or at least that is what vaccine-makers claim.

Residual agents include bovine serum (a popular agent used to grow the virus in cell cultures); formaldehyde (used as an inactivating agent); and antibiotics such as neomycin, streptomycin and polymyxin B to prevent bacterial contamination.

Animal Products: Animal products are most frequently used in vaccine production as the medium in which the virus is cultured and grown. They perform two essential functions: they provide nutrition to the pathogen and they provide cell lines that help it replicate to make the millions of doses that are then commercially sold.

Animals whose organs, tissues, blood and serum are commonly used to make vaccines are monkeys, cows, sheep, chickens, pigs and occasionally dogs and rabbits.

Human Products: Human fetal cells (human diploid cells) divide indefinitely and are used to make cell lines that make a virus replicate. For instance, the rubella virus is grown in human tissue culture as the virus is incapable of infecting animals.

After a virus is cultured, the pathogen is purified while removing it from the growth culture. However, traces of genetic material from the culture often remain in the vaccine.

This presents a real and ever-present danger. If the host animal or human being is infected, secondary pathogens are likely to be passed on during vaccination.

This is exactly what happened when the polio vaccine, grown in monkey kidney cells, were later found to be contaminated with the Simian Vacuolating Virus 40 or SV40. (See Chapter 2: Historical Blunders).

Having looked at the broad categories of components in vaccines, here is a list of some toxic agents (with documented side effects) used in their production.

- Acetone: Nail polish remover
- Oil Adjuvants: A neurotoxin linked to Alzheimer's disease and seizures. It can also precipitate arthritis
- Formaldehyde: A carcinogenic agent used as an embalming fluid
- Ethylene Glycol: Antifreeze widely used in car engines
- Triton X100: A detergent
- Glycerin: Can damage internal organs such as the lungs, liver and kidneys and gastrointestinal tract
- Monosodium glutamate (MSG): According to the FDA, MSG Symptom Complex or MSG side effects can result in numbness, burning sensation, tingling, facial pressure or tightness, chest pain, headache, nausea, rapid heartbeat, drowsiness, weakness, and difficulty in breathing for asthmatics. More specifically, studies have shown that MSG can cause arrhythmia, atrial fibrillation, tachycardia, rapid heartbeat, palpitations, slow heartbeat, angina, extreme rise or drop in blood pressure, swelling, diarrhea, nausea/vomiting, stomach cramps, rectal bleeding, bloating, flu-like achiness, joint pain, stiffness, depression, mood swings, rage reactions, migraine headache, dizziness, light-headedness, loss of balance, disorientation, mental confusion, anxiety, panic attacks, hyperactivity, behavioral problems in children, attention deficit disorders, lethargy, sleepiness, insomnia, numbness or paralysis, seizures, sciatica, slurred speech, chills and shakes, shuddering, blurred vision, difficulty focusing, pressure around eyes, asthma, shortness of breath, chest pain, tightness in the chest, runny nose, sneezing, frequent bladder pain, swelling of the prostate, swelling of the vagina, vaginal spotting, frequent urination, nocturia, hives (may be both internal and external), rash, mouth lesions, temporary tightness or partial paralysis, numbness or tingling of the skin, flushing, extreme dryness of the mouth, face swelling, tongue swelling, bags under eyes
- Phenol or Carbolic Acid: A lethal toxin used in household and industrial products as a disinfectant as well as a dye

- Thimerosal (derivative of mercury): A toxic heavy metal used as a preservative. Closely linked to autism, autoimmune diseases and other neuro-developmental disorders
- Aluminum: A metallic element which, besides damaging the brain in children, can also predispose adults to neurological problems such as Alzheimer's disease and dementia
- Polysorbate 80 (Tween80™): An emulsifier that can cause severe allergic reactions, including anaphylaxis. In addition, according to a Slovakian study on rats published in the journal Food and Chemical Toxicology in 1993, Tween80 can lead to infertility. Tween80 accelerated the rats' maturation, prolonged the estrous cycle, decreased the weight of the uterus and ovaries, and caused damage to the lining of the uterus indicative of chronic estrogenic stimulation.
- All this makes me wonder why so many millions of people started to get afflicted with the diseases that are listed as side effects of these toxins after mass vaccinations were introduced into modern societies. Most of these diseases were nearly unheard of before the vaccine-mania began.

8. Vaccine 'Mistakes'

The danger from vaccines doesn't come only from these dangerous ingredients that go into them. There are other grave concerns. Among these are the vast gaps in scientific knowledge that exist in modern medicine. These gaps are then filled by what researchers call 'theories', which become the basis of government policies and even the production of medicines to ostensibly prevent disease.

When these mistakes are 'careless slip-ups' made by pharma companies, lives are lost and many people left diseased and dangerously ill. The fallout of the mad cow disease outbreak and the way it was handled by both governments and drug companies has left a controversial legacy that still affects human lives.

Mad cow disease is also called Bovine Spongiform Encephalopathy or BSE, which was first observed in cattle in the mid-1980s in the UK. It is a fatal neurodegenerative disease, whereby infected proteins called prions invade the brain, spinal cord as well as other tissues in the affected cattle. These prions literally eat away at the soft brain tissue, creating holes that leave the brain tissue looking like a sponge.

Around a decade after the outbreak, in the mid-1990s, doctors in the UK observed a disease in human beings they believed had been contracted by eating beef and other animal products from cows infected with BSE.

The disease was first noticed in 1996 and was deemed to be a variant of a disease called Creutzfeldt–Jakob Disease or vCJD. Since vCJD has a long gestation period of several years, it was presumed that the victims had once eaten beef and other products from BSE-infected cows a decade earlier. The disease had claimed more than 160 human lives in Britain by 2009.

Both mad cow disease and vCJD are types of spongiform encephalopathy. However, to date, science has been unable to prove a causal link between the two. How do we know for sure that vCJD, first described by the scientists who lent their names to the disease back in the 1920s, did not evolve into a new strain independent of the animal variant?

Yet, fuelled by hysteria whipped up by the scientific and medical community, the British government opened floodgates of funding of research into vCJD, a move motivated perhaps more by politics than science.

The World Health Organisation (WHO) itself states that "the hypothesis of a link between vCJD and BSE was first raised because of the association of these two TSEs (Transmittable Spongiform Encephalopathy) in time and place".

It adds: "More recent evidence supporting a link includes identification of pathological features similar to vCJD in the brains of macaque monkeys inoculated with BSE. A vCJD-BSE link is further supported by the demonstration that vCJD is associated with a molecular marker that distinguishes it from other forms of CJD and which resembles that seen in BSE transmitted to a number of other species."

However, if vCJD did indeed arise from 'mad cows', then the consequences may have already proved fatal. The shocking truth is that despite being aware of the risks of using bovine material (tissue, calf serum, cow hide and bones used to make gelatin for virus culture) in the production of vaccines, drug companies in the UK covertly continue to use bovine material to make their vaccines.

An investigation conducted by the British newspaper The Daily Express in May 2, 2000, revealed that seven vaccines were at risk of being contaminated. These vaccines had been administered to millions of children made between 1988 and 1989 and administered until 1993.

Vaccines made by two drug majors in particular were identified:

- MMR (Measles, Mumps, Rubella) vaccine (GlaxoSmithKline)
- Various vaccines for Diphtheria, Tetanus and Pertussis (Wellcome)
- Oral polio vaccine (Wellcome)
- Inactivated polio vaccine (GlaxoSmithKline)

Alarm bells also went off in the US, which subsequently drew up a list of suspect vaccines. The health authorities in the US suspected that the bovine material used to make them had come from countries that were affected by mad cow disease. The list included:

- OmniHIB or flu shots (Aventis Pasteur)
- Combination vaccines for diphtheria, pertussis and tetanus (North American Vaccine and GlaxoSmithKline)
- Havrix hepatitis-A vaccine (GlaxoSmithKline)

The above data illustrates just how governments and policy makers take sweeping decisions based on pure hypothesis and how unscrupulous drug companies knowingly indulge in criminal (mal)practices with no regard for the lives they claim to protect.

At the end of it all, do we really know what's going into that vial?

Chapter 2

Historical Blunders

Modern medicine has tried to convince us (and for the most part pretty successfully) that vaccines are a sort of armor, protecting the human body against repeated attacks from disease-producing germs.

But the reality is quite different, and at times, quite the opposite. The truth is that the genetic and chemical vaccine cocktail has been shown to *cause* disease and even *accelerate* its spread.

When we study and analyze the historical record of the many pandemics that have killed large swathes of the population across continents, it makes you wonder how many lives could have been saved, had hundreds of thousands of people not been vaccinated at all.

When you read the following information, there are several factors you might want to bear in mind. Vaccination research has always been a cutting-edge area of medicine, and mass immunization provides researchers, drug companies and governments a captive and willing human sample to test new drugs and formulations.

Introducing these chemicals into the human body through vaccines sometimes has little or nothing to do with the vaccine being administered or the outbreak of a particular disease. In other words, throwing ethical considerations to the wind, researchers have used mass vaccinations as a readymade testing ground or a human laboratory, as it were.

On other occasions, scientific ignorance and inadequate equipment and testing procedures have led to errors of judgment in the development of vaccines, which has cost thousands of lives while leaving others afflicted with debilitating diseases.

In still other instances, either the antigen, or the contaminants, or the additives in vaccines have actually caused disease and death.

1. The Polio Controversy

It is not surprising then that more than half a century after the first polio vaccine was developed, controversy still rages over the contamination of the vaccine with the deadly SV40 virus.

The Simian Vacuolating Virus 40 or Simian Virus 40 is found in the kidney cells of the rhesus monkey. The SV40 is carcinogenic, causing tumors especially sarcomas or cancer of the connective tissue.

Let's rewind to the mid-20th century, when polio was a health crisis across continents and had claimed more than 50,000 lives in the US alone. No wonder the development of the first polio vaccine by Dr Jonas Salk ('dead' or Inactivated Poliovirus Vaccine or IPV) in 1953, and the second polio vaccine ('live' or Oral Polio Vaccine) by Dr Albert Sabin in 1957, were embraced with a collective sigh of relief.

Mass vaccinations began as soon as the Salk vaccine was approved by federal agencies in 1955, and by 1961, more than 90 million people across the globe were inoculated with the IPV.

But it took only two years after the Salk vaccine was approved for scientists to discover that it contained strains of SV40, which lives in the rhesus monkey's kidney cells (the rhesus monkey's kidney cells had been used to grow the polio virus). In subsequent years, numerous eminent scientists and research studies confirmed this contamination after demonstrating that SV40 could infect and cause cancer in human cells.

More recently, the *American Journal of Medicine* cited many studies which have reported the presence of SV40 from the polio vaccine in human brain tumors and bone cancers, malignant mesothelioma, and non-Hodgkin's lymphoma.

In the late '50s, when the SV40 controversy could no longer be ignored, the United States Food and Drug Administration (FDA) decreed that companies submitting their polio vaccines for approval to the FDA after June 30, 1961, must be free of SV40 contamination.

But the FDA left two gaping loopholes for drug companies. One, the government allowed vaccine manufacturers who had made millions of doses prior to June 30, 1961, to sell their vaccines till their shelf life expired two years later.

Two, the FDA did not require vaccine-makers to discard tissue cultures and other related material. What some vaccine manufacturers claimed to have done to prove that their vaccines passed muster after 1961 was to add rabbit anti-SV40 antibodies to their viral cultures to neutralize the simian virus!

With drug companies keeping their facilities under lock and key, there is no way to officially prove that they actually did this. Also, the assumption that these rabbit antibodies were effective against the SV40 has never been proved. Also, vaccine manufacturers have never been forced to prove that they had indeed destroyed their contaminated stocks worth millions of dollars.

Despite this charade, four decades after the first polio vaccine was developed, the World Health Organization proclaimed in 1994 that it had eradicated the scourge of polio from the face of the planet.

However, the damage had already been done. In a candid admission, the US Centers for Disease Control (CDC) announced that around 10-30 million Americans may have been inoculated with the SV40-contaminated IPV whereas another 10,000 people may have been administered the OPV. What the CDC omitted to mention was that millions of individuals in the former USSR, where clinical trials on the OPV had been conducted, had also received the vaccine.

Here is another way to present the argument that the polio vaccine does not produce immunity. If live viruses in vaccines can still induce polio today when standards of sanitation and hygiene are high, it is plausible to assume that the polio epidemics half a century ago were also caused by immunization against the disease when hygiene, sanitation, housing and nutritional standards were relatively crude. What is absolutely clear is that the infection rate is high in areas with poor hygiene. It is important to know that only 0.1 percent of all polio infections are likely to progress to paralysis. The rest of symptoms resemble other viral infections such as influenza.

No matter what may have caused polio outbreaks in the past, it is ethically, morally and medically questionable today to immunize vast sections of the population against a disease that scarcely exists any more but may be experience a comeback because of mass vaccination.

2. Vaccines Cause Disease

There is more than sufficient evidence to show that vaccines have repeatedly failed to prevent disease. In fact, history is littered with instances where vaccination during epidemics has actually led to an increase in the incidence and further spread of the diseases they were meant to prevent and eradicate.

Yet with statistical manipulation and pro-vaccine propaganda, the medical fraternity has been able to convince most of us that these chemicals protect the human body from disease and death.

After the polio controversy, let us learn another lesson from history. Smallpox had been sweeping across 19th and early 20th century Europe and taking a heavy toll, till Britain finally passed a law mandating compulsory and universal smallpox vaccination in 1854.

It was a disastrous mistake. In the years following 1854, every successive smallpox outbreak coincided with a mass vaccination campaign. In other words, there was a sudden increase in the incidence of the disease after the vaccine was administered to the population en masse.

The London epidemic (1857-1859) claimed more than 14,000 lives; the 1863-1865 outbreak resulted in 20,000 deaths; and between 1871 and 1873, smallpox spread across Europe, recording the worst epidemic of the disease in history. In England and Wales alone, the disease claimed 45,000 lives despite the fact that 97 percent of the population had been vaccinated by then!

Germany too experienced the same vaccination pains. The country had passed a law allowing for compulsory vaccination in 1834. Yet, as the disease raged across England, Germany too took a heavy hit.

Despite a rigorous vaccination campaign that had covered 96 percent of the population, the country recorded 125,000 deaths from smallpox. Of these, 17,000 cases in Berlin took place among a fully-vaccinated population. Baffling, isn't it?

But Europe alone has not suffered the mistakes of history. Compulsory vaccination against smallpox in 1872 in Japan caused a spurt in the disease every year after that, till the country registered 165,000 cases and 30,000 deaths in 1892. Ironically again, most of the victims had been vaccinated against smallpox.

Compulsory vaccination was introduced in the Philippines in the early 20th century, which seemed to result in a marked decline in smallpox in that country. However, inexplicably, the disease dealt a deadly blow between 1917 and 1919 in an epidemic that saw 160,000 cases and 70,000 deaths. Here too, the population affected had been fully vaccinated.

There may be several reasons why the smallpox vaccine didn't work then, the most frightening and real one being that the very premise on which the smallpox vaccine is based is flawed.

The smallpox vaccine is made from the genetic material present in cowpox, a disease in cows characterized by pustular lesions on the animal's udders. Incidentally, it was the cowpox virus – or vaccinia virus – which lent its name to the generic term 'vaccine'.

Though vaccine manufacturing procedures are refined today, the smallpox vaccine is still made from the vaccinia virus, and though the scientific establishment today publicly denies this, its so-called success is based on pure presumptions rather than scientific experimentation.

These presumptions were made by an 18th century English physician named Edward Jenner, who had observed that milkmaids and farmers who worked with cows infected with cowpox appeared to be resistant to smallpox.

Jenner went a step further and experimented with the cowpox and smallpox viruses on human beings. In 1796, he injected the smallpox virus into an eight-year-old boy who he had already inoculated with cowpox and observed that the child did not die. (!) Jenner then proclaimed that his 'theory of vaccination' was successful.

This and other 'experiments' performed by Jenner, all of them based on loose observation, managed to convince the medical establishment then that he had found a vaccine for smallpox.

What if it wasn't the cowpox that had produced immunity but the human immune system that prevented Jenner's 'subjects' from developing smallpox? The English physician's 'proof' that the vaccine did indeed work was to round up farmers who had contracted cowpox and inject them with material from smallpox lesions. When the farmers showed no symptoms of smallpox, Jenner offered this as 'proof'.

What if these farmers had already acquired immunity to smallpox from exposure to the disease from others infected with it? When others presented cases that suggested exactly the opposite, Jenner's defense was to scoff at these claims!

Half a century later, England and the rest of the world were to pay for Jenner's unscientific and incredible claims.

Vaccination history continues to expose the claims and myths of global bodies such as the WHO and the Red Cross, who have spearheaded immunization programs across the world. Yet, in a huge embarrassment for the WHO, Ghana was declared measles-free by the global health agency in 1967, after a mass immunization drive that covered more than 90 percent of the country's population.

The WHO should have been more careful before making such bold and self-congratulatory statements because between 1970 and 1972, Ghana was hit by one of its worst-ever measles outbreaks. The *Journal of Tropical Pediatrics* reports that 235,930 cases were recorded during that period including 834 deaths.

Measles outbreaks and immunization programs continue in Ghana today, turning history's mistakes into a billion-dollar industry for the drug companies who make these vaccines.

The claim that the measles vaccine protects against measles is totally unsubstantiated. Although most Japanese children are vaccinated against measles, a measles outbreak took place in Japan in April 2007, causing a total estimated 27,600 cases.

The US is far from immune to the tall claims made by the pro-vaccination lobby. In 1989, measles outbreaks were reported in American schools where 98 percent of the children had already been vaccinated. These outbreaks were recorded across geographies.

The American Medical Association admitted in 1990 that despite the fact that 95 percent of school children are covered by mass vaccination campaigns against measles, it has failed to altogether stop the disease. The incident sparked a heated debate, with some researchers claiming that immunization suppresses the immune system, leading to a general vulnerability to infection.

The case for the spread of diseases by vaccines becomes iron-clad when you include whooping cough, tuberculosis and diphtheria and practically any other communicable disease.

In a bold move, Sweden decided to stop inoculating the population with the whooping cough vaccine in 1979 when the country discovered that of the 5,140 cases which surfaced in 1978, more than 80 percent had been vaccinated three times already.

The New England Journal of Medicine reported a study conducted in 1994 which found that more than 80 percent of children aged under five who were afflicted with whooping cough had already been inoculated against the disease.

In the UK, the Community Disease Surveillance Centre detected more than 200,000 cases of whooping cough in children between 1970 and 1990. All these children had already been vaccinated.

Returning to polio, *after* the introduction of mass immunization. in the US in 1955, the number of polio cases increased by 50 percent between 1957 and 1958, and by 80 percent from 1958 to 1959.

In five states, cases of polio doubled after the vaccine was given to large numbers of people. As soon as hygiene and sanitation improved, *despite* the immunization programs, the viral disease quickly disappeared.

3. Oops! We Forgot!

There are several conclusions we can draw from the data presented above. Foremost among these is that history has established no causal link between vaccination and protection from disease.

The immune system is the most critical factor that determines whether an individual develops a certain disease or not. It is also a factor that was not taken into account during the development of vaccines.

All that these pioneering researchers noted was the prior presence or absence of the disease in the individuals they observed while conducting their experiments. There were no long-term studies (and still aren't) and no control groups used.

Other crucial factors that contribute to the development and spread of are living conditions. Poor quality living conditions, overcrowding, unsanitary and unhygienic environment and malnutrition, and most importantly, vitamin D deficiency due to lack of regular sun exposure, systematically weaken the immune system, thus compromising its ability to maintain homeostasis and ward off disease.

It is no coincidence that epidemic outbreaks have declined over time as the quality of living improved. By that same yardstick, diseases take a far greater toll in poorer countries where malnutrition, contaminated water and unhygienic conditions are widespread.

A glaring omission while performing a headcount during an epidemic or tallying the death toll is that the medical establishment has never stopped to inquire into the medical histories of the individuals affected by the 'killer' virus in question.

Despite this, during epidemic outbreaks, the polio, smallpox and whooping cough viruses, among others, are routinely blamed for cases whose weakened immunity may not have saved them from most illnesses anyway. This raises serious questions about the very foundation of vaccine theory and the so-called efficacy of vaccines.

This is also a matter of documented record. A study conducted by the British Association for the Advancement of Science reveals that improved hygiene and sanitation between 1850 and 1940 coincided with a 90 percent decline in childhood diseases in general.

In the US, the Metropolitan Life Insurance Company documented the four leading causes of death from infectious diseases between 1911 and 1935. It named diphtheria, scarlet fever, whooping cough and measles.

By 1945, the death toll from these diseases had fallen by a dramatic 95 percent – before the advent of mass immunization programs for these diseases. Again, this dramatic decline in disease was due to improved sanitation, nutrition and better housing.

Buttressing the argument for hygiene leading to decrease in mortality, is the CDC's *Morbidity and Mortality Weekly Report* of July 30, 1999, which cites better sanitation, water quality, hygiene and the introduction of antibiotics as being the most important factors in disease control in the 20th century.

Could it be that these advancements (with the exception of antibiotics which weaken the immune system) were boosting health and immunity and saving lives, and not vaccines? The descending and ascending timelines for disease and better conditions, respectively, coincide almost too perfectly to ignore this conclusion.

But when it comes to vaccination, there are more sinister factors at work – the deliberate manipulation of facts to suit the ulterior motives of the medical establishment and drug companies. This includes fudging data, misdiagnosing disease, under-reporting a disease in patients who have been vaccinated against it and over-reporting illnesses in patients who have not been afflicted by them. All this to support the theory that vaccines save human lives!

4. The Semantics of Disease

One of the most obvious factors that affects the incidence – or apparent incidence – of an infectious disease is its definition. And history has shown how sleight of hand, or a few strokes of the pen, can seem to make diseases appear, disappear or look less menacing.

In the US, during trials of the Salk vaccine, there appeared to be a significant decline in the number of polio cases between 1954 and 1957. But did you know that the definition of polio was rewritten during that period?

By this single stroke of genius, the number of polio cases was destined to fall during this crucial time – specifically chosen because the Salk vaccine was officially approved in 1955, when mass vaccination was introduced. It was a deliberate attempt to suggest that the new vaccine was responsible for the decline in the infectious disease.

The medical community took three steps to ensure this. One, diseases that had hitherto been misdiagnosed as paralytic polio were now suddenly excluded from the definition of the disease. These diseases included viral and aseptic meningitis, which had been affecting thousands of children in the US annually.

While the medical establishment may have corrected an inaccuracy, doing so at this juncture served the agenda of the promoters of the polio vaccine. Conversely, in a double sleight of hand, cases of non-paralytic polio were now being classified as viral or aseptic meningitis!

As if this was not enough, an overzealous medical establishment was intent on bringing down the apparent incidence of the infectious disease even further. It therefore raised the limit for the declaration of an epidemic from 20 to 35 for every 100,000 people. This meant it required a larger number of cases to declare that the disease had assumed alarming proportions.

The definition of polio was overhauled in one more critical way. To qualify as polio, symptoms of paralysis had to now persist for 60 days as opposed to just 24 hours. Convenient, isn't it?

5. Hiding The Virus

Medical records are replete with examples of how statistics have been twisted to suit hidden agendas. One way to do this is to conceal the whole picture. Take a bunch of medical statistics out of context and you could get a drastically distorted view of infectious diseases.

Here is an example of how this was done by two researchers from the University of British Columbia, Vancouver, in the book Communicable Diseases Handbook. Arguing in favor of the red measles vaccine in the US, the authors claim that inoculating the population with the vaccine (80 million doses) post-1963 brought down the number of cases from 500,000 before that year, to around 35,000 in 1975.

Nothing wrong with these figures – till you read them against the pre-1963 figures for red measles or rubeola. In 1958, there were 800,000 rubeola cases, indicating that the number of cases was actually falling before the vaccine was administered in 1963.

Add to this picture figures for 1955 and you will see that the death rate for red measles had already fallen 97 percent since the early 1900s!

All this hoopla when there was a bigger lie being perpetrated on the American public in the '60s. The CDC publicly admitted that the inactivated vaccine for rubeola administered between 1963 and 1968 was ineffective, and advised the public to get re-vaccinated! So was the massive drop of red measles infection that occurred between 1963 and 1968 due to the ineffective vaccine, and the continued reduction of infections after 1968 due to the effective vaccine after re-vaccination?

Here is another way in which the medical fraternity has hoodwinked not only the public but budding researchers as well. Close scrutiny of medical texts and journals will reveal that infectious diseases across the spectrum appear to decrease in incidence and severity from 1940 onwards.

Is it any coincidence that this was also the time when advances in antibiotics were made and many immunization programs were undertaken? Deliberately excluding data that reflects the incidence of disease before the era of mass vaccination suggests that vaccines are the champions of good health.

However, medical students, fed on a distorted picture of disease and on baseless assumptions, therefore regard their textbooks as the absolute truth and thus, over time, medical untruths turn into 'fact'.

Here is another example of a dishonest medical establishment. According to publicity material published by a provincial government in Australia, a three-decade-long campaign against tuberculosis before the 1950s had considerably whittled down the incidence of the disease in the country.

Again, even a quick look at statistics from the 1920s reveals that the disease was already in decline well before drugs were introduced to combat tuberculosis in the country. The march of modern medicine had, in fact, little if anything to do with the situation. Alas, they are always quick to usurp credit.

So do infectious diseases pose any significant threat to us now? Well, see for yourself. According to Dr. Robert Sears, author of The Vaccine Book, the number of childhood cases of diseases included on the vaccine schedule in the US in 2007 was:

- Pneumococus – approx. 10,000 cases a year
- Diphtheria – 5 cases per year, 0 cases some years
- Tetanus – 1 case per year in children under 5
- Pertussis – approx. 10,000 cases a year
- Hepatitus B – 30 cases in 1 year olds, 30 cases in 1-5 year olds
- Rotavirus – 500,000 cases, 50,000 hospitalizations, 20-70

- deaths
- Polio – 0 cases since 1985
- Measles – 50-100 cases a year
- Mumps – 250 cases a year
- Rubella – 250 cases a year
- Chickenpox – 50,000 cases a year
- Hepatitis A – 10,000 cases a year, most in children aged 5-14
- Flu – Millions of cases
- Meningococcal Disease – approx. 3000 cases a year

To reiterate, vaccination has nothing to do with these low infection rates. Improved sanitation, nutrition, healthcare and living conditions played a major role both before and after vaccines came on the scene. Other first-world nations, such as Iceland, which give just a third of the number of vaccines to children than the US, experience the same decline in infectious diseases as every other country that improves living conditions.

However, the vaccine fraud comes tagged with a hefty price to pay. In the US:

- 1 in 6 children is diagnosed with a learning disability
- 1 in 9 children suffer from asthma
- 1 in 94 develop autism
- 1 in 450 become diabetic

Vaccinating – or rather poisoning – millions of children one shot at a time, year after year, leaves us with future generations that have to live with disabilities and chronic diseases. We are literally breeding sick populations for many years to come, until hopefully, some day, vaccines will be banned because they are largely being considered responsible for the continuously escalating healthcare crisis.

Switching Diseases

When the term 're-diagnosis' is used by the medical fraternity, it spells 'hoax'. Re-diagnosis, or changing diagnostic criteria, is usually a means to falsify statistics to achieve a pre-determined objective. And the pro-vaccination lobby uses it time and again to support the premise that vaccines work.

According to the National Anti-Vaccination League in Britain, more than 3,000 fatal chickenpox cases were reported in England between the turn of the century and the 1930s. The league goes on to point out that chickenpox is not a fatal disease and that the deaths took place due to smallpox. Doctors had allegedly 're-diagnosed' smallpox cases as chickenpox because each of the individuals affected had already been vaccinated for smallpox.

Remember, the smallpox vaccine was the 'first successful vaccine ever to be developed'. Hence, the re-diagnosis served to cover up the embarrassment of the medical establishment.

Chapter 3

Is There A Conspiracy?

Part I: WAR ON INFANTS

The history of vaccination is littered with so many inaccuracies – and doctoring of medical records – that it is sometimes hard to sift fact from fiction. No matter how much has been written or spoken about the efficacy of vaccination, the truth is that there is absolutely no proof that vaccines work.

Later in this book, we shall discuss the absolute lack of scientific studies to prove that vaccination theory is founded on sound scientific principles. Suffice to argue for the time being that if it indeed were, the medical establishment would not need to distort figures and present selective data to prove that vaccines are effective.

Alternatively, a theory founded on scientific fact does not need propagandists as it speaks for itself.

So who benefits from brainwashing the public with such untruths? What are they trying to hide? What are their ulterior motives? Just how do they achieve their devious ends?

1. Modern-Day Pogrom?

As we debate these ethical and moral issues, we shall also take a look at the often-lethal consequences of these unconscionable actions. Not surprisingly, some researchers and anti-vaccination campaigners go so far as to compare immunization campaigns to Nazi 'pogroms'.

Why else would Western public health agencies thrust a polio vaccine on Uganda when the African country did not have a history of the disease? (More on this in Part III: All The World's A Lab). If the anti-vaccine camp has been accused of exaggeration and paranoia, their beliefs seem to gain credibility as you delve into the details. With increasing awareness and access to information, thanks to tools the Internet and other technologies have given us, evidence is piling up, for instance, to make a convincing case that AIDS was deliberately introduced to Africa by Western governments.

What better way to control entire nations than by keeping them sick, weak, impoverished and at the mercy of donors?

There are powerful material benefits to controlling entire nations, not least of which are their abundant natural resources like oil. Is it too farfetched to believe that vaccination is being used as a deliberate means to manipulate, scare and even kill people in nations where lack of literacy subdues the will of the people and discourages them from asking 'awkward' questions?

When the Oral Polio Vaccine (OPV) was introduced to Nigeria in 2002, Muslim clerics rallied the population to revolt. The campaign was born of skepticism of Western nations and their motives.

Whether justified or not, there were suspicions that the OPV contained infertility agents targeted at Nigeria's Muslim population. Some reminded UNICEF, which was spearheading the polio immunization campaign in Nigeria, of the horrific clinical trials conducted by American drug giant Pfizer in 1996.

The Nigerian government has since sued the company, which was then experimenting with an antibiotic drug called Trovan. The drug was administered to 233 Nigerian children with bacterial meningitis during an epidemic. During the clinical trials, 196 children died and the remaining 37 children suffered debilitating health problems including paralysis and brain damage.

The third reason the Nigerian population was outraged by UNICEF's polio vaccination campaign was the accusation that the Western world, through agencies such as the World Health Organization (WHO) and other global non-profit bodies, had deliberately introduced HIV to Africa in the 1950s through the polio vaccine. The vaccine was administered to a million people in what is now Rwanda and Burundi, where the earliest cases of HIV in Africa were later detected.

Whether true or not, there is widespread skepticism in several quarters regarding mass immunization campaigns and the seemingly altruistic intentions of international public health and aid agencies and their motives. Is it all conjecture? (More on this in Part III: All The World's A Lab and Chapter 4: Critical Mass)

2. Who Stands To Gain?

All this suggests a medical conspiracy of sorts, involving the pharmaceutical industry, the medical establishment, health regulators and policy-makers. If this were true, what's in it for these vested interests?

The truth is more layered than is immediately apparent. While only some – a core group – can be accused of consciously and deliberately plotting the murder of innocent children and adults, there are many who collude unwittingly.

At the core of the vaccine cartel are pharma companies, senior members of the medical fraternity, policy makers and health regulators. Drug companies earn billions of dollars a year from the sale of vaccines and research grants while politicians have their own ulterior motives.

But, pray, why would someone as lowly in the pecking order as, say, a general practitioner, push the same agenda? Surely, he or she can't be in on a global conspiracy?

Let me put it this way. Why are diseases that result from vaccination misdiagnosed so very often? Is there a deliberate attempt to cover up the truth? What has the doctor to gain by hoodwinking a child and his or her parents?

When a doctor brought up in the fine traditions of allopathic medicine is confronted by glaring discrepancies, it is a natural tendency to rationalize the truth. That is, if a doctor is confronted with a patient who displays symptoms of, say, polio, and he knows the patient has been vaccinated against the disease, he would rather misdiagnose the symptoms than acknowledge that the vaccine did not work, or even worse, that the vaccine actually caused the disease.

Why would doctors stake their reputation and fundamental beliefs on a system of medicine by questioning the very basis of their life's work? Unconsciously or not, generation upon generation of medical practitioners and specialists have thus, and in many other ways, pushed the cause of vaccination. They were simply raised to do so during years of academic study.

Others may indulge in pro-vaccination propaganda and even fudge clinical data to secure coveted and lucrative research grants and fellowships, public recognition and awards.

Just as the motives are many, the players in this dangerous game of smoke and mirrors are also many. But the objective is always the same: to conceal the truth from the public.

It is a closed system that works on many levels, a system that has worked perfectly for the last 200 years since Edward Jenner 'developed' the smallpox vaccine, also touted as the world's first 'successful' vaccine. (The modern version, Dryvax made by Wyeth Laboratories, was approved by the US Food and Drug Administration in 1931)

3. An Ignorant Public

But a system such as this works only if we buy into it. And we have. The most oft-used tactic used by the vaccine lobby is fear. Leveraging this primal human emotion and burned into public consciousness is the fear of 'dire consequences' (read death) if we don't vaccinate our children, ourselves and even our pets!

It is a message that comes to us through subtle and blatant advertising paid for by pharma dollars to perpetuate the myth that vaccines protect our health and save human lives.

Mass hysteria is another extremely effective tool, witnessed most recently during the 2009 swine-flu outbreak and before that the SARS outbreak in 2002. This pandemic of fear, fuelled by an overzealous media, enabled the vaccination of millions of willing and unwilling victims across many continents.

What were in those vaccines? Were researches using the hysteria to test unknown strains of viruses and chemical additives? Was the global pandemic deliberately engineered? (See Chapter 7: *Swine Flu: The Pandemic That Didn't Pan Out*)

Another weapon to brainwash a willing public is the media, which sold out to corporate pharma decades ago. How often we read about the "successful" results of public health agencies such as the WHO every time an immunization campaign is conducted! Such propaganda serves only to reinforce the so-called life-saving nature of these lethal cocktails. How often do we read about wonder drugs written about by a media whose owners often have close ties to Big Pharma?

Finally, public ignorance has also helped perpetuate the notion that vaccination is a rite of passage that every child must undergo in the first few weeks of their lives. The brainwashing (regarding the benefits of vaccination) begins in the maternity ward. It continues in school, and as we grow up, we are bombarded with public service messages on the need for immunization.

It's a crafty tool as education and public service messages are 'positive' and do not create resistance. They effectively create a certain mindset, which makes the public easily vulnerable to other tactics such as fear and mass hysteria.

Finally, the human tendency for quick-fix solutions and an easy way out completes the cycle of brainwashing. For most people, it's easier to submit to a couple of jabs than live a healthy lifestyle and boost one's immune system the way nature intended.

Living healthy is often hard work, considering the way modern lifestyles are designed. But instead of investing in healthy nutrition, adopting healthy sleeping habits, exercising, and spending time in the sun to make us immune against most diseases, we prefer to vaccinate ourselves and our children.

How easy it is to turn an untruth into sound scientific theory – in the case of vaccines, it's taken just 200 years.

4. Sudden Death

Sudden Infant Death Syndrome or SIDS is a convenient term the medical establishment has coined to describe deaths in infants resulting from an inconclusive diagnosis. It is a convenient term that conceals the number of infants who actually die of adverse reactions to vaccination.

The only official estimate comes from the Vaccine Adverse Effects Reporting System or VAERS cell sponsored by the Centers for Disease Control (CDC) and the Food and Drug Administration (FDA). VAERS records the reports of vaccine-related reactions as well as deaths in infants submitted by the public and doctors when vaccination goes wrong. However, few are aware of VAERS and few doctors use the system. Here is a quote from the VAERS website:

"More than 10 million vaccines per year are given to children less than 1 year old, usually between 2 and 6 months of age. At this age, infants are at greatest risk for certain medical adverse events, including high fevers, seizures, and Sudden Infant Death Syndrome. Some infants will experience these medical events shortly after a vaccination by coincidence. These coincidences make it difficult to know whether a particular adverse event resulted from a medical condition or from a vaccination. Therefore, vaccine providers are encouraged to report all adverse events following vaccination, whether or not they believe the vaccination was the cause."

VAERS's statistics reveal that on average, doctors in the US report 11,000 cases of serious vaccine-related events every year. Of this, 1 percent of infants die after being vaccinated. That's approximately 100 children a year.

If these figures appear low, consider the FDA's own estimates – that doctors report only 10 percent of vaccine-related *serious* adverse reactions (hospitalization, life-threatening illnesses and permanent disability) to VAERS. Hence, the number of infant deaths reported every year – approximately 100 – is actually infinitesimal.

No matter how much the medical community cloaks the truth, researchers agree that SIDS is linked to vaccination. According to one independent study, the number of SIDS cases in the US is greatest in infants aged two to four months, which is when babies receive the first round of vaccines. Other studies have found a three-week lag between vaccination and death.

While none of these studies can conclusively state that vaccines killed these infants, it is difficult to draw any other conclusion considering the weight of research that correlates the two variables. You may also recall that in countries like Iceland where children receive less than a third of the number of vaccines given to children in the United States, the death rate is also 50 percent lower.

Interestingly – and alarmingly – VAERS data reveals that a large portion of the reported "adverse events" pertain to vaccines for pertussis or whooping cough, a disease routinely 'taken care of' by the DPT vaccine (Diphtheria, Pertussis and Tetanus). Independent studies state that children die eight times faster than normal after a DPT shot.

Considering the extent of underreporting to VAERS, it is difficult to estimate how many individuals are seriously disabled by vaccination. One estimate, quoted during a lawsuit, claimed that one in every 300 DPT immunizations causes seizures.

It was in response to widespread concerns over the DPT vaccine that the US Federal Government set up the National Vaccine Injury Compensation Program, loosely called the 'Vaccine Court', to settle claims against vaccine manufacturers in cases of adverse reactions to their drugs.

Since the NVICP was set up in 1998, it has received 5,000-odd claims including 700 pertaining to vaccine-linked deaths. The total sum awarded in compensation to date is $724 million.

5. Early Assault

Despite the overwhelming evidence that vaccines are not safe and that there is no conclusive evidence that they protect us from disease, we consent to allow these harmful chemicals to be pumped into our children.

On the contrary, there is a growing body evidence to suggest that vaccines may, in fact, thwart a child's immune system from developing normally. For instance, doctors have found that individuals who have not suffered a bout of measles in childhood are more prone than those who have, to skin diseases, diseases of bone and cartilage, and certain types of tumors. It has also been found that individuals who do not contract mumps are more prone to developing ovarian cancer.

Some researchers believe that the viral genetic material in the chickenpox vaccine may surface years after vaccination in the form of herpes zoster or shingles or other disorders of the immune system.

Confirmation of this trend is seen in the increase of adult shingles by 90 percent from 1998 to 2003, following the release of the chickenpox vaccine for mass use. Shingles is linked with three times as many deaths and five times as many hospitalizations as chickenpox.

Chickenpox has never been a serious illness, at least until 1995 when the live virus chickenpox vaccine was licensed in the United States and mass vaccination began. Before and even now, for 99.9 percent of healthy children, chickenpox is a mild disease without complications. Children who have chickenpox by age six develop a natural, long-lasting immunity to it.

After Merck developed and distributed the chickenpox vaccine in 1995, chickenpox was suddenly declared a life-threatening disease for which children must get vaccinated or face serious health problems!

By vaccinating and thereby preventing children to develop natural immunity to chickenpox, we are now facing a new epidemic of adults getting shingles. Chickenpox is caused by the varicella zoster virus, which is a member of the herpes virus family and is associated with herpes zoster (shingles).

After recovering from chickenpox, the virus can remain dormant in the body's nerve roots for many years, unless it is reactivated. Physical or emotional stress and exertion are among the most common activators. When awakened, the symptoms present themselves as shingles rather than chickenpox.

Nature creates chickenpox to strengthen natural immunity and prevent shingles. Children who go through the disease naturally and later come into contact with other children recovering from it receive a natural immune booster which helps them to stay protected from contracting shingles later in life. In other words, by not allowing chickenpox to occur in the population of children, we are risking an epidemic of shingles among the population of adults. We have been taught to stay away from people who are infected with chickenpox. In truth, if you have already had chickenpox in the past, coming in contact with someone who has chickenpox actually serves as a further 'booster vaccine' to help avoid shingles, regardless your age.

Since the mass-introduction of the chickenpox vaccine, there is just not enough chickenpox around to keep providing natural immune boosters to children and adults. Hence the man-made escalation of shingles among adults.

Shingles, marked by pain and a blister-like rash on one side of the body lasting three to five weeks, does not typically lead to serious complications. However, in persons with a weak immune system (which happens after being vaccinated), complications may be serious and even life-threatening. These include postherpetic neuralgia, bacterial skin infections, Hutchinson's sign, Ramsay Hunt Syndrome, motor neuropathy, meningitis, hearing loss, blindness, and bladder impairment.

As it often happens, the short-term benefits achieved through the silver-bullet approaches of medical intervention, actually lead to irreparable disasters in the long-term. Accordingly, we may have achieved a decline of chickenpox (mild illness) among children through mass vaccination, while having generated a near-equal increase of shingles (severe illness) among adults.

Please note that the chickenpox vaccine may only provide temporary, superficial immunity, whereas recovering from chickenpox bestows long-lasting superior immunity. According to the Centers for Disease Control and Prevention (CDC), "The effectiveness of the vaccine is 44 percent against disease of any severity and 86 percent against moderate or severe disease." I am not sure how they can know this for sure, especially since their estimates underwent major revisions in recent years.

Investigations of a recent chickenpox outbreak in a New Hampshire daycare revealed that it began with a child who had previously been vaccinated. And as reported by the Washington Post, in another outbreak, 75 percent of the affected children had been vaccinated against chickenpox.

It also helps that most 10-year-old children are naturally immune to chickenpox even though they have not gone through the illness. A Canadian study involving over 2,000 school children found that 63 percent of youngsters with no history of chickenpox had antibodies against the virus. It is presumed that they had a very mild case of chickenpox, which produced no symptoms at all, or just a runny nose and a mild rash. In fact, most infections (of any kind) are uneventful, and we will never know that we were infected. In other words, it is very beneficial for children to hang out with other children who are recovering from chickenpox.

Of course, the same principle works for adults. Researchers at Britain's Public Health Laboratory Service (PHLS) found that adults living with children enjoy higher levels of protection from shingles.

We must remember that we have a smart immune system that doesn't require us to fall ill to become immune to most illnesses. Just breast-feeding for at least one year is known to bestow children with the most effective immune system there can be.

In any case, it may be a blessing that the chickenpox vaccine is as ineffective as it appears to be. This may actually prevent an even more serious shingles epidemic than is already in the making. However, this blessing in disguise may be short-lived. The drug giant Merck has already developed a shingles vaccine (Zostavax) to help foil the escalating shingles epidemic which it helped to create by disseminating its chickenpox vaccine. Approved by the FDA in 2006, the vaccine is being targeted at people age 60 and older, at the cost of $200 a shot, and regardless whether these older folks are already immune-compromised or suffer from another illness such as cancer. For the medical industry it's just another clever marketing scheme. First, they cause the problem and then they offer their help in fixing it. The fix, in turn, causes even more health problems, which then require new fixes. And so the medical Ponzi scheme continues to grow exponentially.

The main question here is whether it is worth risking the health or life of your children, now or in the future, for no real benefit at all. Consider the following adverse events that may accompany chickenpox vaccination:

According to the federal Vaccine Adverse Events Reporting System (VAERS), between March 1995 and July 1998, one in 1,481 chickenpox vaccinations were followed by an adverse health event.

Among the adverse events, about 1 in 33,000 doses involved serious complications such as shock, encephalitis (brain inflammation), thrombocytopenia (a blood disorder) cellulitis, transverse myelitis, Guillain-Barré Syndrome, and shingles.

Fourteen out of the reported 6,574 chickenpox vaccine adverse events ended in death.

Given the fact that adverse vaccine events are notoriously underreported – by as much as 90 percent – the more probable 140 deaths instead of the reported 14 cases should caution every parent and doctor about such a risky vaccination program.

The risk may be even greater when the vaccine is combined with other vaccines, like MMR, which was confirmed by Barbara Loe Fisher of the National Vaccine Information Center (NVIC). She said: "We have been getting reports from parents that their children are suffering high fevers, chickenpox lesions, shingles, brain damage and dying after chickenpox vaccination, especially when the vaccine is given at the same time with MMR and other vaccines."

The bottom line is, vaccination offers no advantage over non-vaccination. Vaccination only helps to further increase the incidence of disease and thereby generates an endless requirement for medical attention, which in turn benefits those who make money off the unsuspecting population.

This brings us back to the issue of natural immunity versus acquired immunity discussed in Chapter 1: The Vaccine Myth. In other words, childhood infectious diseases gift the body with a natural immunity that vaccines purport to artificially induce, but in vain.

The fact is that we are assaulted by pathogens – bacteria, viruses, amoeba, etc – every single day but do not succumb to the infectious diseases that these germs are alleged to produce. This is solely due to the body's immune system and other natural filters that continuously and tirelessly kill and weed out non-beneficial germs and debris every single day of our lives. Individuals whose immune system has been compromised and who are unable able to keep their insides clean require an invasion and proliferation of germs to help detoxify their bodies for them.

The immune system consists primarily of white blood cells, antibodies and the lymphatic system. White blood cells and lymph circulate throughout our organs, tissues and cells while simultaneously cleansing them of cellular debris, toxins and naturalizing pathogens along the way.

That's not all. The immune system is beautifully layered and operates at various levels. It is also composed of various lines of defense that a pathogen must encounter so that it can effectively deal with the pathogen. In other words, the body uses multiple filters while screening for pathogens to make sure anything that is harmful

50

perishes before it can cause an infection, unless, of course, an infection becomes warranted and the body allows it.

What are these various 'filters'? In addition to the already mentioned mucus lining along the body's orifices, saliva protects against germs and our skin serves as armor for our internal organs. The liver is the body's supreme filter and purifier, and cleanses the blood of all types of toxic waste including chemicals and by-products from drugs as the blood passes through the organ.

Then there are the excretory organs such as the kidneys and the large intestine and bowels to get rid of solid waste. When you breathe out, the air you exhale too contains cellular waste just as your perspiration does.

The fact is that in order to create natural and real immunity to disease, a pathogen must provoke the complete inflammatory and immune response. This is a complex response that resonates throughout the body's equally complex immune system. When this happens naturally, the body acquires life-long immunity to a particular germ.

But for this to happen, the pathogen must pass through natural channels, from outside to inside. For instance, the pathogen must pass from the respiratory system or through the saliva or skin and then to the other organs involved in filtering it out such as the mucus membranes, thymus, liver and spleen.

Vaccines do not do this. Instead, they completely bypass the outside-to-inside process by being directly injected, thereby failing to provoke the full immune response.

By injecting a live but attenuated virus, parts of a virus or a dead virus, vaccines trick the immune system into releasing antibodies against a particular pathogen. This shortcut, as it were, is what vaccine theory is based on and is seriously flawed.

For instance, it was only later discovered that the immune system is composed of two parts. While one part is active, it suppresses the other part and vice-versa. Artificially stimulating one part of the system to produce antibodies abnormally inhibits the other part of the system and thus throws the entire immunological response out of gear.

One of the major repercussions of this is that the body sometimes begins to produce antibodies that attack its own cells, thus creating an autoimmune disease. At least that's the theory behind such autoimmune disorders; but I will offer a slightly different explanation below. The organ that is affected depends on which tissues are attacked by the antibodies.

For instance, when the brain and spinal cord are attacked, the individual develops vaccine-induced encephalitis. This in turn leads to a number of diseases including Guillain-Barré Syndrome and other neurological diseases that often manifest themselves in behavioral symptoms.

Is it pure coincidence that the incidence of autoimmune diseases such as rheumatoid arthritis, asthma, minimal brain disorder, autism and subacute lupus erythematosus has increased dramatically as the medical establishment recommends multiple-vaccine immunization?

Indeed there are other factors that cause autoimmune diseases but some researchers are unequivocal that vaccines are also responsible. In my opinion, it is not the antigen itself, but the foreign protein particles and chemical additives in the vaccines, such as mercury, aluminum, formaldehyde, body parts containing foreign DNA, and squalene that produce the same response.

Once this toxic sludge is injected directly into the blood, it will inevitably make its way into the brain, spleen, kidneys, liver, joint fluids, blood vessel walls, lymph vessels and connective tissues of intestines, lungs, breasts and other parts. The multiple tissue damage caused by these toxins requires a continuous and significant healing response by the body that includes the production of antibodies. As already mentioned, the body uses antibodies to heal damaged tissue and neutralize accumulated harmful toxic substances. To successfully detoxify and heal the affected tissues, antibodies and other cells of the immune system must inflame them first.

An overreaction of the immune system may occur when the body becomes overwhelmed with the sudden appearance of unnatural, toxic substances in the blood such as mercury and antibiotics. Modern medicine conveniently calls such a healing attempt autoimmune disease, meaning, the body attacks itself. In truth, the body has no intention to commit suicide.

Let us now see how vaccines contaminate the immune system and why they throw it off-balance. Most vaccines are 'live' vaccines i.e. they contain the intended virus, which is weakened so that it doesn't produce full-blown symptoms of disease, before it is introduced into the human body.

Before that, the virus must be 'cultured' or grown artificially while being fed on nutrient-rich substances such as aborted human fetuses, chick embryos, pig embryonic tissues, and monkey kidney cells.

Can you imagine how putrid this 'culture' must be? The next step is to remove the impurities and isolate the virus by subjecting it to a series of complex chemical processes.

When the attenuated or weakened virus is introduced into the human body, the body by reflex attempts to neutralize the intruder and produces a greater amount of antibodies in the process. This is a violent biochemical reaction as under normal circumstances, viruses rarely if ever enter the body directly through the bloodstream.

Yet, vaccines contain chemical additives called adjuvants to exaggerate the initial immune response. They also contain chemical fixers to stop the immune system from altogether destroying the antigen. Destroying the viral material would defeat the very purpose of the vaccine, right? Next, preservatives are added to the vaccine to prevent it from putrefying and to create shelf-life.

Among the chemical additives in vaccines are monosodium glutamate, thimerosal (mercury), antibiotics, anti-freeze and other acidic and toxic compounds.

Children are the most vulnerable section of the population because their immune systems are practically defenseless against these poisons. They have a lot against them since most mothers were once vaccinated and hence fail to pass on their own natural immunity to them through breast milk.

More evidence that vaccines are lethal to children comes from James R Shannon of the National Institutes of Health. He said, "No vaccination can be proven safe before it is given to children."

A new life, whose immune system is already compromised, cannot effectively cope with such a genetic and chemical assault. According to an Australian study, children who received the pertussis vaccine were five times more likely to contract encephalitis from the vaccine than developing encephalitis by contacting pertussis through natural means.

Also, when babies are immunized, there is no regard for the infant's unique biochemical make-up. Since babies scarcely have a medical 'history', there is no way to tell what medical vulnerabilities the infant might have. For example, a prematurely born child is typically not as healthy as one that was born at full-term.

Still, vaccines are administered regardless of individual differences (the same applies to older children and adults). It's a one-dose-fits-all policy. Also, doses are not varied with body weight and other variables.

As soon as the vaccine is administered, the infant's body musters all its strength to eliminate it. If the child is biologically sensitive or weak, the vaccine may pass through the crucial blood-brain barrier and damage the brain's cells. Autism is just one of the many debilitating neurological consequences of vaccination.

In the section that follows, we shall further explore how vaccines declare an all-out war against the human immune system.

Part II: THE WAR WITHIN

If scientists, policy makers and pharma companies have turned myth into 'scientific truth' for two centuries, here is another fact that is alarming, to say the least. Scientists including virologists and the lay public simply do not know enough about vaccines.

There are too many gaps in scientific knowledge to justify administering vaccines to infants or to adults; government policies give vaccine-makers (and drug companies in general) the privilege to conceal details of their formulations, testing procedures and data behind an impenetrable curtain of secrecy.

There are contamination issues the public will never know about (SV40 contamination in the polio vaccine is only the tip of the iceberg). And pharma companies all too often make mistakes and then 'voluntarily recall' batches of their vaccines.

1. Fatal 'Errors'

The tragic death of Baby Alan Yurko in 1997 documents what can happen due to sheer carelessness by doctors and Big Pharma. Baby Alan died two and a half weeks after he was born.

The infant had been given six vaccines, including a one dose of the Diphtheria. Tetanus & Pertussis vaccine (DTaP). The vaccine had been administered despite contraindications for DTaP, which advise against vaccination in babies with any type of infection or premature births. Baby Alan scored on both counts apart from having other vulnerabilities passed on by his mother, all of which are listed as contraindications for vaccination.

Baby Alan's records state the cause of death as Shaken Baby Syndrome or SBS (whose symptoms closely resemble those exhibited by the infant), for which the infant's father was charged, even though doctors later admitted that the case had been misdiagnosed.

Among Baby Alan's symptoms were swelling of the brain, hypercoagulability of the blood, inflamed blood vessels and subdural hematomas, all of which also result from violent and repeatedly shaking an infant as in SBS.

Subsequent research has revealed that many cases thought to be SBS are actually vaccine-related deaths, which could have been avoided, had physicians administering the vaccines stopped to check the babies' medical history.

There was one other shocking truth about Baby Alan's death. The DTaP vaccine he was given was later found to have come from what vaccine-makers call a 'hot lot'.

These are batches of vaccine that have an undue number of vaccine-related 'adverse events' associated with them, as the potency of the vaccine is much higher than intended. By definition, a 'hot lot' is a batch of vaccines that is too potent and can potentially infect recipients with the disease it was meant to protect them from!

In other words, these are lots where something has gone drastically wrong during the manufacturing process and are recalled as and when the errors are discovered, often too late.

Further investigation into Baby Alan's case found that the DTaP dose he was administered came from the 'hottest lot' of the vaccine (made by Connaught Labs). This is substantiated by the fact that an unusual number of infants died after being given doses from this batch, between 1990 and 1999.

Despite the revelations from Baby Alan's case, there have been more infant deaths from vaccines that were improperly manufactured. All this because vaccine-makers are not really concerned with human life and this amounts to blatant medical negligence.

Clearly the medical community and vaccine manufacturers had not learnt a lesson from the Tennessee 1979 'crib deaths', a catch-all phrase that was used to conceal the fact that 11 babies, all of them administered a DPT vaccine made by Wyeth Laboratories, had died of vaccine-related complications. (Note: DTaP is a safer version of an older vaccine called DTP which is no longer used in the United States)

The 'Tennessee Cluster', as it was also called, sparked a furor and the CDC was obliged to order an investigation which included inputs from the US Surgeon General's Office, the Tennessee Department of Health and the FDA.

Not surprisingly, despite the testimonies and assistance of numerous noted doctors and medical consultants from various American Universities as well as major drug manufacturers, the Tennessee crib deaths were officially never recorded as vaccine-related.

In fact, in an article in the *Journal of Pediatrics* (1982), the chief investigator appointed by the CDC, Dr Roger H Bernier, was quoted as saying his panel could neither find a causal relationship between Lot # 64201 and crib deaths although it could not exclude one either.

Sitting on the fence was convenient for everyone and it covered Bernier's own position as well.

Independent investigations later revealed that the vaccines administered to the 11 Tennessee infants had come from a 'hot lot', whose potency was *double* of what was it should have been.

The vaccine was so potent that all 11 babies had died after the first shot itself. After the Tennessee tragedy, vaccine manufacturers learnt a lesson – they have since changed their distribution practices. Lots are now scrambled to avoid 'clustering' and detection should a 'hot lot' make its way into the commercial supply chain!

Scrutiny of medical records reveals that the DTaP shot and its variants are associated with an unusually high number of vaccine-related adverse reactions. These include brain damage, convulsions, abscesses and allergic reactions. It is the component of the vaccine that is supposed to protect against pertussis (the 'P' in DPT) that is most dangerous.

2. Vaccine Recall

When a vaccine (or any drug for that matter) is recalled, what happens to it? Vaccine-makers are not saying anything. Insiders and whistle blowers suggest that they are ploughed back into circulation. Also, scrambling doses to avoid the detection of 'hot lots' reduces to near-zero the chances of adverse reactions drawing attention.

Here are some recent cases of vaccine recall recorded by the CDC.

* In December 2009, Sanofi Pasteur voluntarily recalled four lots of its H1N1 pediatric vaccine because the antigen content was below the "pre-specified" potency limit.

In case you're wondering how small a 'lot' is, read this: The four lots made by Sanofi Pasteur totaled a staggering 800,000 doses of the H1N1 virus. The company admitted that the vaccine was 12 percent less potent than it should have been even though it has insisted that the vaccine had been thoroughly checked at the time of manufacture. How then did the potency drop? And what about the thousands of children who had already received the vaccine?

The company's official position was that the vaccine was still strong enough to protect children against the H1N1 virus! Count the number of possible loopholes and the scenario raises alarm bells.

Sanofi Pasteur was not the only vaccine maker who had slipped up on the H1N1 vaccine. In December 2009, AstraZeneca announced that it was recalling its H1N1 nasal spray vaccine, MedImmune, for the very same reason: lowered potency. The defective lot involved 4.7 million doses, most of which had already been shipped out for commercial use.

Of course, the drug maker issued a disclaimer, claiming that the vaccine was at full potency when it had left the company. Oddly enough, they also claimed that recipients of the vaccine need not re-vaccinate themselves. So why recall the drug?

* In July 2009, Wyeth recalled one lot of its Prevnar pneumococcal 7-valent Conjugate Vaccine for diphtheria because, by its own admission, the lot in question was not meant for commercial use. The company admits that the syringes containing the vaccine were "inadvertently" mixed with those meant for commercial sale.

We still don't know what went out in those doses and whether recipients of the vaccine from this lot could suffer fatal consequences.

* In December 2007, Merck recalled 13 lots or 1.2 million doses of its PedvaxHIB and COMVAX vaccines due to "lack of assurance of product sterility". Hiding behind this seemingly benign term was Bacillus cereus, which causes food poisoning. It had crept into the vaccine from unsterilized (dirty) equipment at one of the drug maker's manufacturing units.

* In 2001, Merck was forced to halt production of two vaccines – the MMR vaccine and the Varicella vaccine for chickenpox – after the FDA found that the facility producing them had failed to comply with certain regulations.

* In October 2006, Novartis recalled two lots of Fluvirin (an influenza vaccine) because it noticed some shipments containing the vaccine in a 'frozen state' or below the required temperature. The company pointed a finger at its distributor.

* In April 2004, Aventis Pasteur recalled one lot of Imovax Rabies, an anti-rabies vaccine, after it discovered that one lot (which it claimed had not yet been shipped) contained a non-inactivated strain of the rabies virus!

All this leaves several disturbing questions unanswered. Not only are vaccines extremely harmful to human health, there isn't enough control over what vaccine-makers claim they're putting into their vials, syringes, oral doses and nasal sprays.

Drug companies aggressively state that they maintain no less than rigorous standards during the manufacturing processes. How then can they account for the need to recall their products – repeatedly?

3. Insider Secrets

We talked about contamination in (See Chapter 2: *Historical Blunders*) and the furor created by the discovery of SV40 in the polio vaccine. But it turns out that contamination is fairly common.

As far as pharmaceutical companies are concerned, data and laboratory practices are classified information and it is only once in a while that they become public knowledge.

There is one man who can perhaps shed light on some of the goings-on in the 'sterile' confines of pharma laboratories. He's a vaccine researcher who worked in the laboratories of major drug companies in the US for several years. Now retired, he had also once worked with the US government's National Institutes of Health.

According to him (his identity has been withheld for obvious reasons), we know that a host of biological contaminants find their way into various vaccines. Either drug companies are unable to detect them or they are unable to isolate and remove them. Either way, these contaminants can lead to crippling as well as fatal consequences.

According to the retired researcher, acanthamoeba, a type of amoeba that feeds off brain cells, has been found in the polio vaccine. Acanthamoeba is naturally occurring but is also often found lodged in the kidney cells of monkeys.

What is its connection with the polio vaccine? Monkey kidney cells are routinely used to produce the polio vaccine and if laboratories are not checking for its presence, the amoeba can pass into the vaccine unnoticed.

Acanthamoeba produces various symptoms such as a stiff neck, headaches and fever. Once the amoeba travels to the brain, it damages the organ, which shows up as hallucinations and other behavioral changes.

In fact, there are many types of amoeba that are found to contaminate vaccines. The effects usually manifest in infants as encephalitis and respiratory infections. These microorganisms enter the vaccine either from lab furniture and equipment or directly from the tissues of animals such as monkeys in whose tissues the virus is cultured and grown.

Other monkey viruses that routinely contaminate vaccines are the simian cytomegalovirus, simian foamy virus and the bird-cancer viruses, the latter found in the MMR (Measles, Mumps, Rubella) vaccine.

Bacteria, viruses and parts of these pathogens including the toxins they produce in addition to carcinogenic protein molecules find their way one way or another into the syringes, drops or nasal sprays that contain vaccines which we are told will provide us immunity from dangerous infectious diseases.

Are all of these contaminants dangerous? The truth is, no one really knows. By that same reasoning, is it safe for a vaccine to contain something that cannot be accounted for and whose effects on the body are unknown?

4. Vaccine Time Bomb

There are lots of things vaccine-makers and the medical establishment won't tell you. One of these is the danger – actually, many dangers – that arise from attenuated viruses.

Vaccines that use live viruses (as opposed to those that use an inactivated or 'dead' pathogen) basically contain the live virus of the disease it is meant to keep at bay.

It is supposed to achieve its objective by weakening the virus by adding chemicals such as formaldehyde (See Chapter 1: *The Vaccine Myth*) and by using inactivating agents during the manufacturing process.

The attenuated virus is meant to provoke an immune response that is sufficient to produce antibodies to the virus (but not the full-blown disease), and these antibodies, in turn, are meant to protect the individual should the same type of virus actually invade the body later on.

However, 'infecting' the body with a live virus, even if 'attenuated', could produce disastrous results. Remember, even if weakened, the virus is not dead and it is circulating in the body.

Viral shedding is one such consequence. It is a process whereby a vaccinated individual spreads the live attenuated virus through excretion via nasal droplets, saliva, urine and feces. This usually takes place for a few weeks after the vaccine is administered.

The virus could therefore spread to family members, classmates, colleagues at work or just about anybody. If the virus, through the sanitation system or any other means, finds its way into the water supply system, the entire community could be at risk. And it could take just one such individual to spark an outbreak among those who already suffer from a pre-existing condition or weak immune system.

Several types of vaccines use attenuated viruses, with flu vaccines, varicella (chickenpox) and the OPV most likely to result in viral shedding. In fact, this was among the many reasons why the OPV was pulled off the market in the US. Some researchers have also found that the rubella virus can be passed on to infants through breast milk!

In March 2009, a New York resident sued Lederle Laboratories, who manufactures Orimune, an OPV. The plaintiff was awarded $22.5 million by a New York jury after he claimed that, thanks to viral shedding, he was infected with the polio virus while changing his baby's diapers. He claimed he had contracted the virus through a wound on his hand and had suffered from polio for 30 years before he filed his lawsuit.

There are other dangers of using attenuated viruses in vaccines, another compelling one being that they wreak havoc on individuals who have a compromised immune system. Among those especially vulnerable are individuals afflicted with autoimmune diseases such as rheumatoid arthritis, AIDS or even diabetes.

The question is whether individuals in this category are allowed to refuse vaccination? What if the state mandates that a certain target population must be vaccinated?

The 2009 swine flu outbreak, which saw forced vaccinations, is a case in point, especially since no one checks individual case histories during mass immunization campaigns or performs tests to see whether a recipient's body may be immunologically weak or compromised.

Take this reasoning one step further and most of the population is at risk because most of us have compromised immune systems thanks to the type and number of pollutants we are regularly exposed to, the pesticides and insecticides in our food, and all the toxic components in the processed foods we eat.

Then there is the question of attenuated viruses evolving into mutant strains. Researchers have documented cases where viral mutants have evolved from vaccines introduced through vaccination, thereby creating and potentially spreading a new disease while attempting to protect against a known one.

This is precisely what happened in Nigeria during mass immunization with the OPV in 2002 and 2006. Paralyzed Nigerian children are still paying for this mistake.

Several research studies discussed in the medical journal, *Lancet*, have noted cases where the Hepatitis B vaccine has also been a notorious culprit. These studies quote findings where infants have developed mutant HBV virus strains, with one study claiming that 3 percent of such babies host a mutant virus and exhibited symptoms such as active liver disease.

In the 1960s, outbreaks of pneumonia from mutant viruses were observed in US soldiers who were tested with a viral pneumonia vaccine.

I want to emphasize that the body responds to viruses (foreign protein particles) that enter the body via the natural orifices, versus the route of injection, in entirely different ways. Injected viruses enter the blood along with potentially life-threatening chemicals, a route for which the body can never properly prepare itself. To mop up the deadly chemicals, the body may require viral reproduction. To help break down damaged, weak cells, the body may require a bacterial infection. The resulting disease is a healing crisis (the attempt to rid the body of toxins and to heal the damage they caused).

Pneumonia is not a disease, but an appropriate and effective approach by the body to trap the circulating blood contaminants in the lung tissue and mucus membranes, and to allow bacteria such as *Streptococcus pneumoniae* to decompose the damaged or dead lungs cells. The resulting sputum is coughed up, sometimes along with toxic blood, and removed. Once the healing process is completed, the symptoms will subside and the lungs will be healthier than before.

The biggest mistake one can make is to interrupt or suppress the healing through the use of antibiotics, antiviral medication or inflammation-reducing drugs. Complications of such interventions frequently end in death.

5. Whipping Up A Storm

The immune system is a complex and intricate system where each cell and its functions are perfectly coordinated or choreographed. Sometimes, this complex interplay is tripped up and the system spins out of control creating a 'cytokine storm'.

Cytokine storms are extremely dangerous and when they affect the lungs, they are often fatal. They can be triggered by various factors, including flu viruses and weakly attenuated flu vaccines.

A cytokine storm is a process where the immune response is short-circuited, causing an exaggerated and overwhelming response which finally leads to organ shutdown.

To understand how and why this takes place, let me briefly explain what happens when a pathogen such as a virus is directly injected into the bloodstream (which is an entirely different case scenario than when it enters the body via its natural orifices). When this happens, the white blood cells – T cells and macrophages in particular – rush to the site of infection and inflammation and chemically devour the pathogen.

If the pathogen is strong, these specialized white blood cells need to call for additional troops. They release a protein called chemokines to signal other white cells to rush to the site of infection and inflammation.

When this signaling process is disrupted (for instance by certain vaccines), the process spins out of control, creating a fierce and lethal storm of cytokines. This creates an endless loop or a runaway immune response.

Whereas normally, rushing more white cells to the site of an injury or infection eventually heals the affected tissue, in a cytokine storm, the body interprets this as a greater cause for alarm and presses even more cells into action.

As a result, the tissue or organ is flooded with cytokines and eventually shuts down. When this response affects the lungs, abnormal amounts of fluid accumulate in the organ, the airways get blocked, and eventually the victim suffers Acute Respiratory Distress Syndrome (ARDS), lung failure and death. Cytokine storms can also result in multiple organ failure when other organs are involved, such as the heart, liver and kidney.

6. Turbo-Charged Vaccines

The cytokine storm phenomenon is relevant in any discussion on vaccines which contain adjuvants. These are chemicals added to vaccines to turbo-charge them. In other words, adjuvants heighten and exaggerate the immune response to a vaccine immediately after it is administered when the antigen used is a live but attenuated or weakened form of the virus.

This means that you need significantly less vaccine to produce the desired immune response than if you did not use adjuvants. Despite the controversial nature of adjuvants, it is clear why pharma companies use these chemical catalysts in vaccines.

By increasing the vaccine's 'potency', they can even quadruple the number of doses with the same amount of antigen! Hence, by using adjuvants, vaccine-makers can automatically quadruple profits, running into billions of dollars a year.

There are many reasons why adjuvants are dangerous, the most compelling being that science does not know enough about them. Yet drug manufacturers use them on the simple premise that they 'work'.

Interestingly, adjuvants were discovered quite by accident. When vaccine technology was still evolving, drug makers noticed varying levels of efficacy in vaccine doses from the same batch. They later discovered that doses that were more potent had been contaminated by the lab equipment.

Further investigation revealed that oddly enough, under more sanitized and sterile conditions, the same vaccine seemed to lose some of its potency. The amazing thing is that though researchers have several theories to explain why adjuvants enhance the immune response, no one really knows for sure.

The term 'adjuvant' itself was coined in the 1920s by a veterinarian, Gaston Ramon, who noted that horses that were administered a diphtheria toxin produced a heightened immune response if the site of the injection was already inflamed. This inflammation could have been produced by various factors, including tapioca and bread crumbs used by Ramon in his experiments!

Later, alum or aluminum salts were discovered to produce the same result and to date, alum is the only adjuvant licensed for use in vaccines manufactured in the US. It is present, for instance, in vaccines for tetanus and Hepatitis B.

As if the lack of scientific knowledge surrounding adjuvants is not scary enough, recent developments during the 2009 swine flu outbreak set alarm bells ringing due to the possible use of an adjuvant derived from squalene.

Though drug makers deny this, many researchers point out that when used as an adjuvant, squalene produces many debilitating symptoms including autoimmune diseases such as rheumatoid arthritis.

Squalene is an oil molecule that is naturally present in the human body. But in its natural form, squalene is harmless and is even hailed for its antioxidant properties. However, it is not the presence of squalene in the body but the manner in which it is introduced into the body that makes it harmful. When it is injected, the immune system interprets squalene as an intruder and begins to attack it.

Worse, the immune system also begins to attack *all* the tissues in the body that contain squalene molecules, not only the adjuvant. This is how squalene as an adjuvant triggers an autoimmune response.

The squalene disaster most frequently cited in medical journals is the reaction it produced in Gulf War veterans in the 1991 conflict in the Middle East. These soldiers were the subjects of experimental trials on the anthrax vaccine which contained squalene. The adjuvant was called MF59 made by the pharma giant Novartis.

These soldiers later – in many cases *many* years later – developed autoimmune diseases and exhibited symptoms such as memory loss, chronic fatigue, seizures, multiple sclerosis, an elevated erythrocyte sedimentation rate or ESR, systemic lupus erythematosus and neuro-psychiatric issues among other medical problems. Despite a conclusive link to the squalene adjuvant in the anthrax vaccine, the FDA has consistently denied any causal connection. Obviously, they don't want to be seen as playing a major role in causing our troops to fall sick.

In the aftermath of the swine flu outbreak, there was considerable concern in the US over whether the FDA would allow vaccine manufacturers in the country to include squalene in vaccines against this disease as it is widely used in Europe and elsewhere.

Currently Novartis calls its squalene adjuvant MF59, which it uses in its seasonal flu vaccines outside the US while GlaxoSmithKline calls its squalene adjuvant ASO3, which is used in its H5N1 bird flu vaccine.

The closest the FDA came to approving squalene for use against swine flu in the US was when the federal government purchased stocks worth $700 million from both Novartis and Glaxo. This was because the squalene adjuvant considerably reduces the amount of antigen required, and during the H1N1 outbreak the US was afraid it might run out of H1N1 vaccine.

What will happen to these squalene stocks? Will they find their way into commercial supplies – clandestinely or not – in the future? Will the government invoke its Emergency Use Authorization powers to use the adjuvant at some point in the future?

Using squalene in its 'war against the H1N1 virus' could deal the human body a double whammy. Flu viruses are notorious for mutating, and mutating fast, and rendering vaccines made prior to the mutation useless.

What if the H1N1 virus mutates – the scientific term is 'antigen shift' – and also triggers a cytokine storm? Should a mutant flu virus invade individuals or entire populations with H1N1 vaccines containing squalene, it would mean a cytokine storm in individuals who are already prone to autoimmune disease.

If all this seems so much conjecture, how is it that vaccine companies have been allowed to get away with so much guesswork about adjuvants anyway? Without sufficient data, how is anyone to predict the evolutionary path that viruses will take?

Part III: ALL THE WORLD'S A LAB

So what exactly *is* in that vial? It's a question that history has answered, all too often, with shocking details. Not least among these is a development that took place in January 2010, when a researcher who made a 'groundbreaking' discovery about the MMR vaccine was discredited on grounds of professional misconduct.

Then there's the web of deceit that covers up (though every now and then some details manage to slip through) vaccine scams that turn those tiny 'life-saving' drops into potentially lethal weapons.

And not least of all, there are question marks hovering over how the Western governments have tried to vaccinate entire populations or sections of the population into submission.

In this section, we shall explore some of these issues while illustrating how untruths are carefully and conveniently converted into 'scientific fact' to suit the profit and political agendas of various stakeholders in the vaccine game.

1. The HPV Controversy

Remember the 'dirty money' connection uncovered in Texas in 2007? Governor Rick Perry had then ordered in the interest of health that every female six-grader be vaccinated against the Human Papillomavirus Virus (HPV) to prevent cervical cancer.

It was an order that bypassed the state's legislature (See Chapter 5: *Critical Mass*), and the governor's attempt to force the vaccine on children caused outrage among parents as well as watchdog and civil rights groups.

Soon, Perry's 'dirty secret' was out – the decision would have earned millions of dollars for the HPV vaccine manufacturer – Merck – who had gifted large sums of money to Perry for his political campaign.

The nexus didn't stop there. In a sequence of events that reeked of kickbacks and more subterfuge, it was revealed that the governor's chief of staff was a senior Merck employee when the governor was pushing the HPV vaccine. With pressure mounting on Perry, the Texas Legislature eventually passed a law rescinding the governor's order.

It is easy to believe slick political-speak only because we have been brainwashed from the cradle that vaccines are good for health. Had the HPV secret not been discovered, thousands of sixth-graders would have been vaccinated with a chemical cocktail that has been shown time and again to prove controversial.

Interestingly, the HPV vaccine at the center of the Texas firestorm was Gardasil, approved by the FDA in June 2006, less than 12 months before Governor Perry attempted his forced vaccination campaign.

Needless to say, administering it to every female sixth-grader in Texas would have provided a ready market for Merck.

Not surprisingly, controversy has repeatedly followed Gardasil, which its makers claim protects against four strains of the HPV that cause cervical cancer and genital warts. According to the CDC, as of September 1, 2009, 26 million doses of Gardasil had been distributed across the US.

The CDC also states that till that date, its VAERS had received more than 15,000 reports of adverse events, of which 7 percent were serious.

Also, these are merely cold statistics till viewed against the type of serious events associated with the vaccine, and in the short period since it was approved, the vaccine has been linked to cases of young women dying just hours after being administered the drug. The vaccine is also suspected to cause blood clots and strokes and has been linked to the Guillain-Barré Syndrome, a rare and debilitating disorder of the nervous system where the nerves get inflamed and which also causes paralysis.

Some public interest groups state that they have gathered sufficient evidence to link Merck's HPV vaccine to 18 deaths, of which 11 took place less than a week after the women were administered the vaccine. Miscarriages were also frequently noted in women who had received this controversial vaccine.

According to a study whose results were published in the *Canadian Medical Association Journal* in January 2009, researchers in Australia had found that Gardasil had provoked a severe allergic reaction – or anaphylaxis – which can lead to death in some cases. The study concluded that the vaccine is 5 to 26 times more likely to cause such a reaction in young women compared to other vaccines administered to the same age group.

The US Federal government finally sounded a warning about the vaccine in July 2009, with VAERS releasing a report which stated that Gardasil is associated with adverse reactions 400 times more than an anti-meningitis vaccine administered to women in the same age group.

As of September 28, 2010, the Vaccine Adverse Events Reporting System (VAERS) has more than 18,000 Gardasil-related adverse events listed in it, including at least 65 deaths. Clearly, the number of vaccine injuries is rising fast. And these are only the reported cases which amount to an estimated 1 to 10 percent of all cases.

The government report also recommended that Congress "investigate how the vaccine was fast-tracked for approval in the absence of safety data on girls younger than 17". The report therefore raises a serious ethical issue: Considering that Gardasil had only been tested on adult women, what moral right did Governor Perry have to mandate the compulsory vaccination of sixth-graders with this lethal and sometimes fatal chemical?

With the mountain of evidence piling up against this vaccine, Gardasil was dealt another blow, this time from the lead researcher on the team that conducted the clinical trials for Merck. In a confession, since retracted under pressure from the pharmaceutical giant, the researcher confessed that the vaccine loses its efficacy five years after it is administered. Not surprisingly, Merck has been selling the vaccine for $400 a dose!

Moreover, independent research suggests that the HPV naturally leaves the body within two years of infection in 70 to 90 percent of cases. If the immune system can naturally eject the virus and even protect the body from future attacks, why do women need a vaccine against HPV in the first place?

The final twist in the Gardasil story comes from a development in October 2009. This was a red-letter day for Merck because the FDA had approved the vaccine to prevent genital warts in boys.

It was no coincidence that the announcement by the vaccine manufacturer came less than a day after rival GlaxoSmithKline announced that the FDA had approved its own HPV vaccine for cervical cancer!

All the data I have presented above raises some serious ethical questions: The motives of at least one manufacturer in the case of one virus (in this case HPV) have been clearly bared as being profit-driven with no regard for the lives of the young women being coaxed to get vaccinated.

Hopefully, the unfolding Gardasil drama will serve as a deterrent to parents and their children to not so readily submit to unproven experimental drugs like Gardasil that were never tested against a true placebo. We certainly cannot rely on the FDA to protect us against the reckless profiteering schemes of drug producers. Being the watchdog body supposed to safeguard the public's health, the FDA had yet again sold out to a vaccine maker with no regard for its objectives.

Finally, if a healthy human body and immune system can do the job of a synthetic vaccine, is a vaccine against HPV necessary at all?

2. Experimenting in Africa

Uganda: Global public health agencies are watchdogs of public health, saving millions of lives on the planet, with most of their objectives fulfilled in poor and developing countries. That's the message the media has been putting out so successfully that most of us believe it is true. But there are hidden agendas, which often remain concealed. But once in a while, their so-called noble intentions are unraveled, laying bare a shocking reality.

Among these was a web of deceit uncovered by an African radio broadcaster who discovered that mass immunizations with the OPV in Uganda were definitely not intended to save children from the debilitating paralytic disease.

Vaccinations with the OPV – which uses the live virus – began in Uganda in 1963, a country that had no history of polio while the government of Uganda introduced mass immunization at the behest of the World Health Organization (WHO) in 1977.

Kihura Nkuba, the broadcaster, who had studied in England, had returned to Uganda to open a radio station there. But his experiences with the Ugandan people revealed a shocking story. Hundreds of Ugandan children who were being inoculated during government-enforced immunization drives were dying of polio.

In other words, the OPV, quite literally being forced down their throats, was *causing* a disease that had not been present in Uganda till the vaccine was introduced in the 1960s.

Nkuba said that parents, who had made a connection between the vaccine and their children's deaths, would hide in the African bush when government officials and health volunteers came around to administer the OPV. In some cases, children were allegedly dragged out of hiding to be vaccinated.

It was only in 2002 that the penny dropped, when Nkuba made the connection between the discontinuation of the OPV in the US and its introduction in Uganda. The OPV, developed by Dr Albert Sabin in the 1950s and which used the live polio virus, had been banned from use in America because it had been observed to accidentally cause the disease in recipients of the vaccine. The US then reverted to using the Inactivated Polio Virus or IPV.

Instead of discarding vaccines worth millions of dollars, these suddenly useless but dangerous doses of the OPV were being force-fed to children in Uganda!

Nkuba realized another shocking truth – that the vaccine when administered in the US was contraindicated for use in families with a history of HIV. That is because the live virus used in the OPV gave rise to a condition called 'viral shedding'. This takes place, as explained earlier, when a vaccinated individual literally sheds the virus through mucous, feces and other bodily fluids for a period of time immediately after being vaccinated.

Naturally, the OPV was not recommended for use in families where individuals have a compromised immune system. But neither was this practice being observed in Uganda, where HIV was widespread, nor was the information being disseminated among the public. The catastrophe that this caused can only be imagined.

Nkuba went public with his observations on the OPV disaster on his radio station and was subsequently hounded and persecuted. Not surprisingly, his radio station was also shut down by the Ugandan government, which he openly accused of committing mass murder hand in glove with the WHO, UNICEF, United States Association for International Aid (USAID) and CDC.

Nigeria: It is easy to use a vulnerable nation – where illiteracy rates are high, where disease is rampant and where global agencies have projected themselves as saviors of the people – as a human laboratory.

Like Uganda, Nigeria is another country where global health agencies have been accused of abusing the trust of the people, and worse still, of committing genocide. This has resulted in a triple whammy for this African nation.

The country has seen severe outbreaks of polio, and even deaths, ever since Western health agencies began a mass OPV immunization campaign in 2002.

A year after the campaign kicked off, the drive was halted after the local people and Muslim clerics alleged that the vaccine contained material that left recipients infertile.

The WHO resumed immunization, this time more 'aggressively' in 2006, in an attempt to cover as many people as possible. But then, soon after, Nigeria saw the beginning of its worst-ever polio outbreak, leaving 60-odd children paralyzed in 2007-2008 and more than 120 in 2009.

What went wrong in Nigeria? In a secret that cost the US CDC huge embarrassment and worldwide censure, the Nigeria outbreak was finally diagnosed as being vaccine-induced. The polio vaccine administered in 2002 resulted in the development of a mutant strain that was now causing the disease in healthy children who had not been vaccinated earlier.

How was this possible? The 'benevolence' of Western health agencies had placed Nigeria in a Catch-22 situation. Children were contracting polio either directly from the OPV while others were left open to the disease because they resisted immunization with a faulty vaccine!

The implication was that to be protected against the mutant polio virus, Nigerian children should have been immunized with a faulty vaccine. All because the WHO decided to 'dump' a vaccine that had been banned in the US.

Why didn't the agency use the IPV that was being used in the US? One, it saved the vaccine maker millions of dollars not to destroy millions of doses. Two, the OPV is cheap. And three, the OPV can be easily administered by health workers and volunteers, not necessarily doctors. This accounts for the popularity of the faulty vaccine in mass immunization efforts across Third World countries.

But it also left the WHO in another dilemma. Immunization programs in Nigeria had been aimed at the polio Type 2 virus but due to genetic mutation, the outbreaks post-2007 were caused by the Type 1 strain!

To cover up its mistakes and make sure they had not left out any known strain of the polio virus, immunization programs in Nigeria have since included two rounds of vaccination that target Types 1, 2 and 3 of the virus! Could there be a bigger mess?

Alas, Nigeria wasn't the only country affected by the OPV mistake. No less than 12 countries have reported cases of vaccine-induced polio over the last decade. During this time, 10 billion doses of the faulty OPV had been administered to children in developing countries, including outbreaks in the Dominican Republic and Haiti in 2002.

3. AIDS – Man-made Virus?

On January 31, 2010, it was announced that scientists had successfully developed a crystal that could show them just how an enzyme involved in the Human Immunodeficiency Virus or HIV works to help the virus replicate itself inside the body.

This breakthrough, they claimed, would enable them to make better drugs to treat HIV, in particular, drugs made by Merck and Gilead Sciences that block this enzyme.

News reports like these are frequently unleashed by the media, leading a gullible and fearful population to believe that drug and vaccine-makers are continuously getting closer to protecting and saving them from "dreaded diseases".

When statements such as the above come from the media, there is a certain credibility attached to them, which is why media houses are the darlings of multinational drug companies.

The truth is much more sobering than the media would have us believe. According to some researchers, dubbed as conspiracy theorists, some diseases spread by viruses and vaccination programs, might be man-made. Among these, some claim, is the HIV that gives rise to Acquired Immuno-Deficiency Syndrome or AIDS.

Was the HIV virus genetically engineered in laboratories in the US in the 1960s and 1970s? Did the virus jump species from monkeys and chimpanzees in Africa and then find its way to the US? Was the virus latent in the human species decades before it surfaced in 1981?

What I am about to discuss, briefly, may read like a medical whodunit and these conclusions are supported by nothing more than circumstantial evidence. But the reason I mention them is to illustrate that scientific research – including research on viruses and vaccines – is classified as 'top secret' as in the case of HIV.

Why should something that is meant to improve public health be hidden away? What does the government not want us to know? And why? There is a vast chasm between reality and perceived reality, which gives rise to frightening possibilities when we entrust our health, well-being and even lives to policy makers and profit-driven pharmaceutical companies.

It is also true that certain target groups – soldiers for instance – have been used in human experiments to test vaccines without their knowledge or consent. This, coupled with the ulterior motives of vaccine-makers, makes vaccination a very dangerous proposition.

Returning to our discussion on HIV, there has been intense speculation on the origins of the virus, leading some researchers to believe that it was cultured in American labs and found its way into homosexual males through the Hepatitis B vaccine in 1978.

Three years after a Hepatitis B vaccination campaign in certain select groups of people, the world's first full-blown AIDS case surfaced in Manhattan in 1981. Cases of AIDS were soon reported from Los Angeles and San Francisco as well.

But if at all it was lab-made, where and by whom was it genetically engineered? Proponents of this theory point a finger at government agencies such as the National Institutes of Health, CDC, the National Institute of Allergy and Infectious Diseases, and big drug companies including Merck, Sharp & Dohme, and Abbott Laboratories, who have been named as participants in certain highly classified experiments that were conducted on primates and other animals for 13 years before the first AIDS case was reported.

These agencies and companies have all been linked to the Federal government's Special Virus Cancer Program (SVCP) from 1964 to 1977. The SVCP, headquartered at the National Cancer Institute in Maryland, was meant to investigate cancer and involved hundreds of thousands of primates and other animals being injected with various types of cancer-causing genetically manipulated material in research centers across the US and in other participating countries as well.

In 1971, after US President Richard Nixon declared a 'War on Cancer', the SVCP was taken over by the US Army's bio-warfare laboratories at nearby Fort Detrick. The laboratories were rechristened the Frederick Cancer Research Center.

During the SVCP, scientists researched (genetically engineered) viruses that produced AIDS-like diseases in monkeys and chimpanzees, leading to sporadic outbreaks in primate centers across the US. It is suspected that these outbreaks were the result of experimental transfer of the viruses between animals as part of the research.

Some believe that this was the origin of some of the various animal cancer and immuno-suppressive AIDS-like viruses and retroviruses that have since surfaced.

Whether these pathogens were deliberately injected into the human population (as conspiracy theorists claim they were) or inadvertently found their way out of the laboratories through contaminated genetic material used to produce the Hepatitis B vaccine is still not known.

Question: Why does the US Justice Department hold propriety over an issue concerning public health such as records relating to the

Hepatitis B vaccination drive in Manhattan and other US cities in 1978, the same vaccination campaign suspected to have led to the first AIDS cases?

4. Going Retro: Chronic Fatigue Syndrome

Scientists love jargon and drug companies love them even more. That is because the more ominous a virus or disease sounds, the faster people will panic and look to pharma companies for a 'cure'.

One of the favorites of vaccine-makers is the term 'retrovirus', a type of virus discovered in human beings in 1981 (or genetically engineered during the Special Cancer Virus Program [SVCP]).

All viruses need a host cell to replicate. However, a retrovirus gets the host cell it infects to replicate itself. It achieves this by incorporating its own genetic material into the host cell's genetic make-up so that when the host produces new cells, it also replicates more retroviruses.

How does it manage to do this? A retrovirus is a type of RNA protein particle that uses an enzyme called 'reverse transcriptase' that converts its own RNA into DNA in the host cell that it infects. The DNA is then transcribed back into RNA, which is how a retrovirus makes copies of itself. This enzyme is unique to retroviruses.

This is a complex process but suffice to say that retroviruses have been associated with a wide range of immunodeficiency disorders, a condition where the immune system seriously malfunctions. In extreme cases, such as in HIV, the immune system appears to attack itself, leaving patients defenseless against the onslaught of the virus and a host of other potentially infectious agents.

Retroviruses have classically been associated with serious debilitating diseases, especially diseases of the immune system. Vaccine-makers have been accused of wielding the 'retrovirus' weapon for disease mongering, that is, first scaring people into believing that a certain virus causes a specific disease and then offering a vaccine to protect them from it.

In my book, Ending the AIDS Myth, I show that the presence of these retroviruses in persons with severely impaired immune systems is merely a correlation and does not prove that the diagnosed AIDS diseases are in fact caused by retroviruses. To the contrary, I show that the dozens of disease conditions, known as AIDS, are actually behind the breaking up of RNA molecules into the retroviruses known as HIV 1, HIV 2, HIV 3, and so forth.

I am certainly not the only one who believes that HIV is not responsible for causing AIDS.

In 1983, world renowned French scientist Dr Luc Montagnier, had discovered HIV for which he received the Nobel Prize in Physiology/Medicine in 2008. Montagnier is currently director of the organization which he helped found: the World Foundation for AIDS Research and Prevention, a UNESCO (United Nations Educational Scientific and Cultural Organization). He has repeatedly stated that HIV alone cannot cause AIDS. Instead of trying to destroy HIV (which cannot cause AIDS) with costly and potentially dangerous drugs and vaccines, Montagnier recommends measures of good hygiene, balanced nutrition, clean drinking water, and antioxidants such as fermented papaya extract to prevent and cure AIDS diseases.

In the 2009 documentary House of Numbers, which can be viewed at www.houseofnumbers.com, Dr Montagnier states: "We can be exposed to HIV many times without being chronically infected. Our immune system will get rid of the virus within a few weeks, if we have a good immune system." This is how any healthy person deals with any virus. In other words, HIV is a harmless passenger virus that bothers no one, unless the immune system has been compromised by other factors, such as polluted drinking water, poor personal hygiene, poor nutrition, oxidative stress, etc.

I suggest we take it from the world's leading virologist. Experts like him know that it is by introducing simple health measures that has always led to the decline of viral epidemics, and not vaccination campaigns. Montagnier believes this to be also the best approach with regard to other epidemics, including malaria. What applies to HIV/AIDS certainly applies to other presumed virus-induced diseases.

One of the diseases currently being blamed on a retrovirus is Chronic Fatigue Syndrome or CFS. This disorder is characterized by extreme muscle fatigue and an all-round, all-pervasive feeling of tiredness.

To date, scientists have been unable to diagnose the causes of CFS but is it believed to be a disorder associated with immune dysfunction. Patients with this disorder have a much higher level of cytokines circulating in their bloodstream, altered T-lymphocyte numbers and low natural killer-cell cytotoxicity. This makes them susceptible to a wide variety of pathogens and afflicted by the disease symptoms they cause.

Lately, though, several researchers have been pointing a finger at a retrovirus called the 'xenotropic murine leukemia virus-related virus' or XMRV. This retrovirus has been linked to prostate cancer as well as CFS patients.

Research findings published in the journal Science in October 2009 state that the virus was found in 67 percent of CFS patients but in only 4 percent of the general population. This has led to a flurry of media reports citing the study and suggesting that CFS may be caused by the XMRV and that a vaccine may be in the offing. When media reports such as these (usually fuelled by drug and vaccine manufacturers) do the rounds, people tend to ignore the critical 'may be', used as a classic alibi by media houses.

Knowing very well that the general populace usually pays little attention to the question marks and 'maybes' in these reports, the media usually gets away with false propaganda about causal relationships between pathogens and disease.

CFS is a disease associated with a seriously compromised immune system and many patients are also afflicted by prostate cancer as well as a host of other diseases. The problem with CFS is that it may not be a single disorder. Researchers believe it may be a collection of diseases that are in some way linked to each other to produce the constellation of symptoms classified as CFS. How, then, can a single virus be associated with a disease about which so little is known?

The Epstein-Barr virus or EBV was at one time thought to be correlated with CFS. But science is still a long way from understanding CFS and many researchers have since minimized the causal relationship between EBV and CFS. Yet, jumping to conclusions and instantly suggesting 'causes' of diseases seem to be the prerogative of the media and vaccine-makers.

Just as the US study on CFS patients created a stir, another research study, this one in the UK, found that none of the 186 CFS patients studied tested positive for XMRV.

The study, undertaken by researchers at the Imperial College London and King's College London, illustrates just how little science knows about CFS and how important it is that we exercise caution while believing what media reports have to say.

Take the HPV discussed above, for instance. Cervical cancer is caused by various factors. Some researchers say it is not caused by a virus at all. Yet vaccine manufacturer Merck is trying hard (too hard?) to convince the public that HPV is the sole cause of this type of cancer and that it has a vaccine to protect against it!

My question is why are none of these researchers and neither the drug companies nor the governments the slightest bit interested in investigating anything other than germs that could possibly impair a person's immune system? It is a rhetoric question to which the answer is obvious. There is not much money to be made by telling people that they need get rid of their vitamin D deficiency, oxidative stress, poor hygiene, nutrient depletion, and overexposure to toxins, including those contained in vaccines and medications.

We know that heavy metal exposure alone can trigger chronic fatigue symptoms and cause brain injury and dementia. Why is the amount of aluminum in the US rivers and streams now up to 50,000 times higher than permitted by US government regulations? Millions of metric tons of Aluminum oxide and other toxic minerals like barium are being dumped by commercial airlines and fighter jets to form chemtrails, allegedly to achieve climate change and protect us against global warming. It is astonishing to me to still find some healthy people in this country!

And, according to a recent CNN report, 45 million Americans live in poverty and suffer from serious malnutrition. Every doctor knows that malnutrition damages the immune system. Merely including the poverty-stricken who currently cannot afford health insurance in a universal health care program, does absolutely nothing to properly address the causes of their health conditions. This approach just fills the coffers of those who know how to create millions of more patients at the expense of taxpayers and send the country deeper into the abyss of irreversible national debt.

5. Vaccine Research: Faking It!

Vaccine-makers are not known to put conscience before science. Scientific research is replete with examples of dodgy data, clinical trials without sufficient controls, non-representative samples and researchers who either unconsciously or deliberately fudge their results. And, no, vaccine researchers are not immune to these maladies.

The swine flu outbreak of 2009 provides many examples of irresponsible media reportage and drug companies who used an overenthusiastic media to push their vaccine propaganda.

For instance, a reputed news agency quoted 'researchers' who claimed that flu vaccines used by pregnant women were likely to increase the birth weight of their infants. It also claimed that pregnant women who took flu vaccines were more likely to have full-term babies. What next, a vaccine against premature births?

Neither of these studies had used randomized, placebo-controlled study protocols. So how were they allowed to be reported? When a responsible media house (this one was Reuters) makes statements like this, the need to be skeptical about what you read is more pressing than ever.

While on the subject of outrageous claims, here is another absurd one: Individuals who take statin-based (cholesterol-lowering) drugs are "50-percent less likely to die from flu"!

A 'news report' undoubtedly sponsored by the makers of statin drugs, recently claimed that "researchers have provided more evidence that cholesterol-lowering drugs help the body cope with infection".

Further probing revealed that there were no clinical trials conducted and that the so-called conclusions were based on a superfluous 'analysis' of the medical records of individuals who had succumbed to seasonal flu infections.

Without taking any other variables into account, the researchers found that a majority of patients from their 'sample' were taking statin drugs; only 3.2 percent were not.

Conversely, they claimed that only 2.1 percent of patients who were taking statin drugs had died. Since 2.1 percent is about 50 percent less than 3.2 percent, they said that "statin drugs can halve the number of deaths caused by seasonal flu"! A masterful example of statistical jugglery but nothing more than wild claims.

Let me illustrate the almost-incestuous relationship between drug regulators and drug manufacturers, something that has always clouded the clinical trials of new drugs. The European Medicines Agency (EMA) is a body of the European Union that approves the sale of drugs across Europe. If the EMA is meant to safeguard the health of the public at large, why did it give vaccine-maker Novartis the green signal to sell its H1N1 flu vaccine Celtura in Europe even though the vaccine was tested on only a hundred people?

Before I answer that question, here's another disturbing fact: The clinical trial based on which Celtura was subsequently sold in several European countries was conducted by the University of Leicester and University Hospitals of Leicester in England – and was sponsored by Novartis.

Scratch beneath the surface a little more and other skeletons begin to tumble out. The EMA also gave two other swine flu vaccines the go-ahead at the same time – GlaxoSmithKline's Pandemrix and Novartis's Focetria.

With two-thirds of the EMA's funding coming from pharmaceutical companies, is it surprising that neither safety, sample size, control groups nor other scientific measures are concerns for an agency that clears drugs for millions of people across the continent?

Did you know that the EMA pays pharma companies millions of euros in 'fees' for services they perform in evaluating the very drugs the companies themselves make?

When pharma, self-serving medical practitioners and the media push the same agenda, it is hard not to be brainwashed. This dangerous nexus between three vaccine promoters – a vaccine technology company, a doctor from Columbia University and the television media – together made a strong case not only for the H1N1 vaccine but vaccines in general in late 2009.

The doctor in question is Dr Mehmet Oz, professor of Cardiac Surgery at Columbia University, no less, an extremely prolific author and vaccine promoter who was on every major talk show during the swine flu outbreak in 2009.

After scaring up a storm on national television, Dr Oz landed a health segment of his own on the hugely popular Oprah Winfrey Show, which virtually launched his television career. After that, he landed a lucrative deal with Winfrey's Harpo Productions and Sony Pictures Television to distribute The Dr Oz Show outside the US, and now it is a popular TV-show in the US.

I have always held a high esteem and respect for Dr Oz because of his continuous effort in making helpful alternative views about many important health topics available to the masses. However, having already been a celebrity doctor for quite some time, I don't understand why he needed to use the 2009 swine flu scare to make millions of dollars from an unsuspecting population.

Soon after his much-hyped Ask Dr Oz segment on TV, it transpired that the doctor owned expensive stock – 150,000 shares – in a vaccine technology company called SIGA Technologies. The company doesn't make vaccines per se but researches and develops technologies used in vaccine production.

Dr Oz's rabble-rousing, it seemed, was almost certainly aimed at driving up stock prices in vaccine companies and vaccine-related companies, which would have earned him – and them – a sizeable booty. During an interview, Dr Oz jokingly remarked that his wife wouldn't allow their children to be vaccinated against the swine flu.

When one comes across instances of deceit and dishonesty like this and stakeholders in a dangerous game colluding with each other, it is hard to tell fact from fiction. A gullible and panic-stricken public is liable to believe what they hear, especially if they're watching 'an authority' on vaccines on one of America's top-rated television talk shows.

Professional ethics took another serious blow in January 2010, when a 12-year hearing on the professional conduct on the doctor who first researched the link between the Measles, Mumps and Rubella (MMR) vaccine came to a close.

The hearing, conducted by the General Medical Council (GMC), the body that licenses and regulates doctors in the UK, ruled that Dr Andrew Wakefield had engaged in professional misconduct.

It was Dr Wakefield's research that had first suggested a link between the MMR vaccine and autism, leading to a furor and declining sales of the vaccine, which had been developed a decade earlier.

While clearly stating that it was not ruling on the authenticity of Dr Wakefield's research findings per se, the GMC concluded that the doctor's methods were blatantly unethical. The most damning revelation was that Dr Wakefield, now residing in the US, was on the payroll of lawyers representing parents who believed that the vaccine had damaged their children's health.

If that was not shocking enough, further investigations revealed that Dr Wakefield had based his findings on a sample of just 12 children! Moreover, the doctor was a gastroenterologist at the Royal Free Hospital in London and was not qualified to perform medical procedures such as lumbar punctures, colonoscopies and MRI scans that he had used in his research.

Dr Wakefield's method of assembling his clinical sample – the 12 children – was equally shocking. He admitted to having bribed them at his son's birthday party to part with blood samples for this research!

The medical journal, Lancet, which had published Dr Wakefield's findings in 1998, issued a retraction of the doctor's paper after the GMC investigation concluded as the doctor had (obviously) not disclosed details of his research methods at the time.

So if Dr Wakefield's original research sparked one of the biggest debates in the area of vaccination, revelations about his professional misconduct have made an impact for quite a different reason.

If Dr Wakefield had been bribed to conduct his 'ground-breaking' research, what about all the other 'ground-breaking studies that are milestones in vaccine research and medical research in general? How many of them have broken the rules? What is authentic and what is not? And how many 'reputed' research studies have been funded by pharmaceutical companies to 'produce' results that promote the vaccines that these companies manufacture or plan to make?

Growing fears that medical research is becoming increasingly dishonest were further substantiated by a study carried out by the University of Edinburgh in June 2009.

The study, published in the peer-reviewed journal PLoS One, reviewed 21 scientific misconduct surveys between 1986 and 2005 and found that faking, falsifying and even fabricating it is more widespread than suspected.

While one in seven scientists surveyed admitted that they were aware of colleagues seriously manipulating their results, 46 percent claimed they were aware of questionable practices by their peers.

Another area of omission is long-term studies on new vaccines. Though researchers know only too well (perhaps because they do) that the side effects of vaccines take months, even years, to surface, they rarely if ever conduct long-term studies to look for possible detrimental effects on the human immune system.

Also, follow-up studies are rarely if ever conducted in vaccinated populations. Most researchers monitor the target group or a sample of it for a couple of weeks only, to detect blatant symptoms.

For instance, symptoms produced by vaccines – such as rashes, arthritis, chronic fatigue, fibromyalgia, memory loss, seizures and neuropsychiatric problems – have a long incubation period as neurological and immunological dysfunctions usually takes a while to manifest themselves.

The icing on the cake for vaccine-makers and drug companies in general is the all-round immunity they enjoy. Regardless of the consequences of the lack of stringent clinical controls, faulty laboratory practices and manipulation of results – and due to their patronization of federal funds, budgets and political campaigns – vaccine-makers are not accountable for their misdeeds.

Thanks to federal laws, they are allowed to keep their formulations and methods secret even while contesting lawsuits, which places a considerable onus on the plaintiff to prove their claims.

Cases against vaccine manufacturers are heard in the 'Vaccine Court' a colloquial term for a tribunal set up under the National Childhood Vaccine Injury Act. The tribunal was established in 1986 to arbitrate the flood of complaints against the DPT vaccine. Ironically, claims are funded by a tax imposed on the sale of every dose of vaccine in the US.

6. Where The Twain Meet

The marriage between medicine and pharma is no accident and dates back to the history of the American Medical Association (AMA), the largest and most influential body of physicians in America.

At a time when the AMA was flailing and near-bankrupt and medical schools in the country were desperate for funding, two of the America's largest philanthropic foundations stepped in – the Rockefeller and Carnegie foundations.

Their funding of the AMA, medical education and sponsorship of the crucial Flexner Report, which brought about widespread changes in medical practices, were a turning point in the history of medicine in the US.

It was a turning point because funding by these foundations was contingent on a certain type of medical education, one that raised doctors on drug-oriented practice. It is these practices – it is no coincidence that pharma companies receive grants from these two foundations – that sowed the seeds of many modern diseases.

The mid-20th century saw another turning point in medicine – the rise of various specialties or branches of allopathic medicine. Suddenly, it seemed, every part of the human body had a specialist to fix it!

This was also no coincidence. The bias towards symptomatic treatment meant that symptoms would recur, which ensured a steady demand for drugs and therefore a readymade market for the drugs made by companies funded by these two foundations.

This was the beginning of a complex web of people and institutions concerned with the medical profession – medical schools, pharmaceutical companies, doctors of all allopathic hues, insurance companies and government health bodies such as the FDA

– seeking in collusion with each other to perpetuate the myth that human health and life lay in the hands of drug makers.

Vaccination is a part of the larger synthetic drug or allopathic myth and therefore the same rules and the same web of deceit apply. So with any immunization campaign or public service message urging the community to get vaccinated, there are ulterior motives. Your health is nowhere on the priority list.

To keep the allopathic myth alive, health authorities have gone all out to discredit any form of medical therapy that is not allopathic. With the help of the media, they and the medical establishment have done a good job of convincing the public at large that drugs – and drugs alone – are insurance for a long and healthy life.

However, in recent years, there has been increasing awareness of these motives and the manner in which the government and pharma companies have been influencing and thus manipulating the public's notion of health and disease.

But is profit the only motive?

7. Hidden Motives

So is profit is the obvious motivator for the vaccine myth? Or are there other reasons why governments immunize vast numbers of the world's population and push the vaccine agenda on an ill-informed public?

The answer to this question is layered and subtle and sometimes hard to digest. The fact is that vaccines target the immune system, cause it to malfunction and make people vulnerable to disease. Sickness ensures a ready market for drug manufacturers and keeps profits rolling in.

But it is not always as simple and blatant as that. Vaccines, believe it or not, also serve subtle political agendas. They help dominate people, groups of people and even countries that the West wants to control – even their own populations. By systematically weakening the people through mass immunizations and predicting a sick fate for those who don't voluntarily choose to vaccinate themselves and their children, governments subtly create a sense of psychological weakness.

This, in turn, creates a sense of powerlessness, submission and dependency on authority figures – government agencies, politicians and world bodies. People are therefore more likely to believe what these 'authority figures' say.

Vaccination is an effective tool used for decades by Western nations, who have sought to exercise social and economic control over several developing countries as clearly illustrated by the African model.

Africa is a continent rich and abundant in natural resources. Keeping the African population weak and preoccupied with sickness and grappling with disease serves Western economic interests. Immunization, along with an influx of economic aid, has worked to effectively subdue possible rebellion and suspend rational thinking.

It's a Machiavellian strategy that involves several layers of people who perpetuate this agenda – UNICEF, the Red Cross, WHO and a mammoth global network of non-profit organizations. And while billions of people are led to believe that their motives are nothing less than noble, vaccines also conveniently channel funds into the bank accounts of specific companies and powerful individuals.

Keeping entire populations or sections of the population sick and vulnerable also diverts attention from real social and economic issues. These issues are inconvenient for governments because they require genuine resolve and huge budgets to tackle.

Academic researchers, reputed authors and some medical researchers also believe that vaccines are being used as a biological weapon to decimate certain socio-economic and ethnic groups. As discussed above, one section of researchers cites the HIV virus as an example of such weapons being designed and engineered in US laboratories to serve this very purpose.

Does this amount to genocide? We are privy to some stunning disclosures by Dr Sidney Gottlieb, a military psychiatrist who held a key position with the US Central Intelligence Agency (CIA) in the 1950s, who later claimed he was instructed by his political masters to use viruses in the struggle for Western control over the Belgian Congo or modern-day Zaire.

In CIA hearings, Gottlieb admitted that he was sent to the Congo with "lethal biological material" (containing viruses), which was to be used to assassinate the country's first elected prime minister after the African nation won independence from Belgium. The country is rich in mineral resources and as soon as it broke free of colonial rule, the US was determined to seize control.

Dr Gottlieb didn't succeed in his mission as the CIA was unable to find a way to biologically poison the politician it was intended for. However, Dr Gottlieb is reported to have confessed in CIA hearings later that he had dumped this "lethal biological material" into the

Congo River. Was he instructed to this or was it an act of carelessness? Some believe it was no accident.

Mass trials of the Hepatitis B vaccine among the American Indian population – whose vast tracts of land have often pitted them against the US Federal government – have also repeatedly raised eyebrows among a section of researchers as well as the American Indian population.

These trials were conducted in 1981 in Alaska, among a people who had no track record of health issues with Hepatitis B. Yet, a plasma-based Hepatitis B vaccine was introduced in schools and in immunization programs among adults as well.

Surprisingly – or not – for school-going children, the program did not require the consent of parents, neither was any justification given for a vaccination campaign among an ethnic community that did not require it.

Several years later – symptoms of vaccine-induced diseases often have fairly lengthy incubation periods – a representation was made before the US Senate Select Committee on Indian Affairs, which claimed that the vaccine may have contained tainted blood that could induce autoimmune diseases in the population.

According to those who made the representation, this was the only explanation for the rise in diseases such as diabetes, cancer and heart disease that were not prevalent among the healthy Native Americans of Alaska.

The representation before the Senate Committee accused the federal government of using the Alaskan population in medical experiments to test dangerous vaccines. It was not the first time such an accusation had been made.

It is a documented fact that certain 'expendable' sections (read ethnic groups) of the human population have been used for medical experiments without their knowledge.

8. Can We Trust Medical Research?

John Ioannidis, who is one of the world's most renowned experts on the credibility of medical research, doesn't think so. According to him and his team of eminent researchers, as much as 90 percent of the published medical information relied on by doctors to prescribe drugs, vaccines or recommend surgery is flawed or incorrect.

In November 2010, *The Atlantic* reports: "His (John Ioannidis's) work has been widely accepted by the medical community ... Yet for all his influence, he worries that the field of medical research is so pervasively flawed, and so riddled with conflicts of interest, that it might be chronically resistant to change, or even to publicly admitting that there's a problem."

In addition, most medical doctors and patients assert that modern medical treatments, including drugs, are "scientifically proven". Not so, according to a *Huffington Post* article (April 2010) by Dana Ullman. "...this ideal is a dream, not reality, and a clever and profitable marketing ruse, not fact". Ullman reports: "The *British Medical Journal's* 'Clinical Evidence' analyzed common medical treatments to evaluate which are supported by sufficient reliable evidence (BMJ, 2007). They reviewed approximately 2,500 treatments and found:

- 13 percent were found to be beneficial
- 23 percent were likely to be beneficial
- 8 percent were as likely to be harmful as beneficial
- 6 percent were unlikely to be beneficial
- 4 percent were likely to be harmful or ineffective.
- 46 percent were unknown whether they were efficacious or harmful"

What's even worse is what happens when doctors hand out unapproved drugs to unsuspecting portions of the population as if they were candy. Ullman writes, "We all want drugs given to infants to be as safe as possible, but mothers and fathers will be surprised and perhaps shocked to know that very few drugs are ever tested on infants." He cites a 2007 study of over 350,000 children which found that a shocking 78.7 percent of children in hospitals are prescribed drugs that the FDA has not even approved for use in children (Shah, Hall, Goodman, et al, 2007). "If this isn't shocking enough, a survey in England found that 90 percent of infants were prescribed drugs that were not tested for safety or efficacy in infants (Conroy, McIntyre, Choonara, 1999)," says Ullman.

This would not be so serious if the treated children were unaffected by these drugs. However, according to Ullman, "there is almost a 350 percent increase in adverse drug reactions in children prescribed an off-label drug than in children who were prescribed a drug that had been tested for safety and efficacy (Horen, Montastruc, and Lapeyre-mestre, 2002)". He says that doctors are committing "medical child abuse" on a regular basis.

These accusations should not be taken lightly by responsible parents, doctors, and scientists. They reflect the serious sickness that medical industry is suffering from, and this sickness affects nearly everyone. The alleged scientific evidence that drugs have a proven value is a myth that has altered the health and quality of life of millions of people, and cost the lives of many others.

Medical science is quackery at its best. As Ullman points out, "'Quackery' is commonly defined as the use of unproven treatments by individuals or companies who claim fantastic results and who charge large sums of money." He says that "although modern physicians may point their collective finger at various 'alternative' or 'natural' treatment modalities as examples of quackery, it is conventional medical treatments today that are out-of-this-world expensive, and despite real questionable efficacy of their treatments, doctors give patients the guise of 'science'."

When over 85 percent of therapies currently recommended by conventional medicine have never been formally proven, we may begin to wonder whether medical science deservers anyone's trust. Would you give your car to a mechanic who offers you a 15 percent guarantee that his minimal mechanical expertise will succeed in fixing a serious flaw in your car's engine? But this is exactly what we do when we hand our lives over into the care of a physician who has been trained by a medical system that is fundamentally corrupt.

The root of the problem is in the way scientific research is being conducted today. For example, during an analysis of antidepressant drug trials, the FDA found that of 38 trials for which the evidence appeared favorable, 37 had been published. Whereas of 36 trials for which the evidence did not appear favorable toward antidepressant drugs, 22 were not published at all, and 11 were published in a way that misleadingly conveyed the outcome as though it was favorable.

Accordingly, drug giants can legally publicize the positive findings they want you and doctors to know about regardless of how poorly 50 percent of the trials reflected efficacy of the studied antidepressant. In others words, the drug makers hide from the public that half of the trials done on the drug failed to prove effectiveness.

Drug makers don't have to publish negative studies. They do as many studies as possible and once they have just two studies with somewhat positive results, they can ignore all the studies with negative ones. There can be as many as 20 negative studies and just 2 positive studies, which is enough for a drug to become approved by the FDA and be pushed on the population. While the positive studies make it into the medical journals, the negatives ones are being pushed under the carpet, never to be uncovered again, unless of course you find an expert on the matter – such as Dr Ioannidis.

In 2005, Dr Ioannidis showed that there is less than a 50 percent chance that the results of any randomly chosen scientific paper will be true. As Dr. Ioannidis wrote: "In this framework, a research finding is less likely to be true when the studies conducted in a field are smaller; when effect sizes are smaller; when there is a greater number and lesser pre-selection of tested relationships;... where there is greater flexibility in designs, definitions, outcomes, and analytical modes; when there is greater financial and other interest and prejudice; and when more teams are involved in a scientific field in chase of statistical significance. Simulations show that for most study designs and settings, it is more likely for a research claim to be false than true. Moreover, for many current scientific fields, claimed research findings may often be simply accurate measures of the prevailing bias."

Again in 2008, in a new analysis published in the *Journal of the American Medical Journal*, Dr Ioannidis reveals that much of the published scientific research is highly questionable. He found that the most misleading studies are those that oversell dramatic or otherwise considered important results. These include articles that helped spread popularity of treatments such as the use of hormone-replacement therapy for menopausal women, vitamin E to reduce the risk of heart disease, coronary stents to ward off heart attacks, and daily low-dose aspirin to control blood pressure and prevent heart attacks and strokes. As we know today, many of these results were falsified, yet millions of people have been (and still are) subjected to these treatments, many of whom were harmed or died. Hormone replacement therapy, for example, led to an unprecedented rise of breast cancers and heart disease, and coronary stents have never shown to reduce mortality from coronary artery disease.

If just 41 percent of the most acclaimed medical research has been convincingly shown to be wrong or significantly exaggerated, which Ioannidis has done in his analysis, the scope and impact of the problem is simply unimaginable. To make matters worse, even after prominent studies were soundly refuted by repeat studies, researchers continued to cite the original results as correct more often than as flawed – in one case for at least 12 years after the results were discredited, according to the analysis.

The main problem is based on the fact that unbiased, independent research is rarely undertaken, lest published. It is very difficult for an independent researcher to raise enough money to fund the research, and if it doesn't stand a chance of becoming published, there is no point spending all that time and money anyway. This unfair selection process ensures that what we are being told is "medical science" is only partial truth at is best. As the saying goes, "a little knowledge is a dangerous thing", we are now collectively and individually facing the consequences of relinquishing responsibility for our own health.

Nearly all major clinical trials involving drugs are funded, at least in part, by drug companies. This makes sense since drug companies have a vested interest in making money off their investment. For example, studies on the world's bestselling drugs, statins, which rake in over half a trillion dollars annually, have all been funded by drug companies. Naturally, drug companies propagated the myth that high cholesterol is our enemy that we must control by taking statins for the rest of our lives.

New discoveries made by researchers at the University of California, published in the *Annals of Medicine* in October 2010, have shown that 92 percent of about 145 clinical trials conducted between 2008 and 2009 are invalid because they didn't disclose the type of placebo they used. By manipulating the placebo, in this case one that actually raises cholesterol in the control group, researchers can easily 'prove' that a statin drug is more effective than the placebo. Read more about this FDA sanctioned medical fraud later on.

Even if the fraud is uncovered and drug companies are fined for manipulating studies or for not disclosing known serious side effects, business continues as usual. Large, publicly traded pharmaceutical companies, like Merck and Pfizer, are simply too big to fail, even if they are found guilty of being the instigators of massive medical fraud. It is unreasonable to expect that any clinical trial conducted by a drug giant procures results unfavorable to their expectations. And yet, drug companies are now the main source to fund the vast majority of research studies in the world. Owning this monopoly on what kind of research is suitable to conduct is what determines our so highly praised 'science-based evidence'.

What we all need to learn from this is whatever drug or treatment is scientifically proven, in no way does it mean that it is safe or effective. Likewise, the lack of scientific evidence that a natural herb or treatment is effective or safe does in no way mean that it isn't. We are responsible for ourselves and our families, nobody else is. I suggest you do your own research and decide what is useful for you and what isn't.

9. Big Pharma on a Rampage

There is more on the scams and frauds in the drug business.

Approximately 200,000 million Americans are killed by prescription drugs each year. There was a time when the common drugs that Americans took were tested chiefly in the US or Europe, but now most clinical trials are unethically conducted overseas in poorer countries where there are next to no regulations; where poor, and often illiterate, people sign on consent forms with a thumbprint; where the risk of litigation is insignificant and where the FDA's supervision is so scarce that the companies have a field day doing as they please. Thanks to globalization, the pharma companies have found new avenues for more unscrupulous money-making.

Romania, Tunisia, Turkey, Estonia, northeastern provinces of China, Poland, Russia - Big Pharma's explorers have been there, and even to remote, isolated towns and locations all over the world to scout out people willing to undergo clinical trials for new drugs, and thus help persuade the FDA to declare the drugs safe and effective for Americans.

Bangladesh has been home to 76 clinical trials, Malawi 61, the Russian Federation 1,513, Romania 876, Thailand 786, Ukraine 589, Kazakhstan 15, Peru 494, Iran 292, Turkey 716, and Uganda 132.

According to the inspector general of the Department of Health and Human Services, until 1990, just 271 trials were being conducted abroad, whereas in a span of less than two decades, in 2008, the number had gone up to 6,458 – an increase of over 2,000 percent!

The National Institutes of Health has been compiling a database and has identified 58,788 such trials in 173 countries outside the United States since 2000. In 2008 alone, according to the inspector general's report, 80 percent of the applications submitted to the FDA for new drugs contained data from foreign clinical trials, and more and more pharma companies are doing all their testing offshore. In fact, 20 of the largest US-based pharma companies now conduct "one-third of their clinical trials exclusively at foreign sites."

All this is happening when 2,900 different drugs for some 4,600 different conditions are undergoing clinical testing and seeking to launch their products into the market.

An important question to ask is: are the results of clinical trials conducted overseas relevant to Americans? People in lesser developed countries may metabolize drugs differently from the way Americans do. Prevailing diseases in other countries, such as malaria and tuberculosis, can distort the outcome of clinical trials.

But the drug companies never had it better, with the cost of running trials far cheaper in such places where the local population just about manages to eke out a living on as little as a dollar a day.

Some of the drugs tested overseas are household names such as the non-steroidal anti-inflammatory drug (NSAID) Celebrex, which has been marketed on television for more than 10 years. Its manufacturer, Pfizer, the world's largest drug company, has spent more than a billion dollars promoting it as a painkiller for arthritis and other conditions, including menstrual cramps.

The NIH maintains a record of most drug trials inside and outside of the US and its database counts 290 studies involving Celebrex, out of which only 183 took place in the US and 107 took place in 36 other countries such as Estonia, Croatia, Lithuania, Costa Rica, Colombia, Russia, Mexico, China, Brazil and Ukraine. It is not mandatory for companies to report all studies conducted overseas, and they make no effort to do so.

So what happened to Celebrex? It was revealed that patients who took Celebrex were more likely to suffer heart attacks and strokes than those who took older and cheaper painkillers. It was also suspected that Pfizer had suppressed a study that drew attention to these facts. No prizes for guessing what Pfizer did next - it denied that the study was kept secret and insisted that it "acted responsibly in sharing this information in a timely manner with the FDA."

Before long, the Journal of the Royal Society of Medicine reported several more negative results. In the meantime, Pfizer was advocating Celebrex to Alzheimer's patients, hoping that the drug would slow down the progress of dementia. It didn't. What did slow down was the sales of Celebrex. From $3.3 billion in 2004, the numbers started declining.

One big factor in the shift of clinical trials to foreign countries is a loophole in FDA regulations: if studies within the US indicate that a drug has no benefit, trials from abroad can often be used in their place to secure FDA approval. When positive data is required by drug companies, and required fast, they turn to seek assistance from the "rescue countries" that quickly come to their aid.

In the 1990s, Aventis Pharmaceuticals (now Sanofi Aventis), developed Ketek, an antibiotic to treat respiratory-tract infections. In 2004, when the FDA certified it effective and harmless, its verdict was essentially based on the results of studies conducted in countries such as Hungary, Morocco, Tunisia, and Turkey. The endorsement came in just a few weeks after a researcher in the US was sentenced to 57 months in prison for forging her own Ketek data. Dr. Anne Kirkman-Campbell, of Gadsden, Alabama, apparently met only willing volunteers to participate in a drug trial. She enrolled more than 400 local adult persons including her entire office staff. In return, she collected $400 a head from Sanofi Aventis.

It was later revealed that data from at least 91 percent of her patients was falsified. (Kirkman-Campbell was not the only difficult Aventis researcher. There were others of dubious reputation as well, but the drug Ketek did win approval on the basis of overseas trials.

Given the massive medical scam operations we are faced with today, including mass vaccination programs, I advice everyone to do their home work before letting those who make a living of defrauding others take advantage of you. The drug giants would quickly turn into harmless dwarfs if we decided to not use their harmful products and fall for their incessant fear tactics, but instead took care of our health in a natural way.

Chapter 4

Critical Mass

Indeed September 11, 2001, was one of America's darkest hours, giving rise to fears of future wars and concerns about bio-terrorism. Post 9/11, the American government consequently passed numerous legislations to put numerous safeguards in place.

So how is America's 'War On Terror' linked to vaccination? That is because among the new and proposed legislations were two that provoked national outrage. Thus from the debris of the Twin Towers came the USA Patriot Act and the Model State Emergency Health Powers Act (MSEHPA), both highly controversial legislations.

While the second is a low-profile legislation, the Patriot Act grabbed the limelight though from the vaccination point of view, both pieces of legislations are equally virulent. I say this because in the interests of safeguarding against terror, the US Federal Government, followed by several American states, have conferred on state governors and other government authorities the power to suspend the people's civil liberties "to control epidemics" and counter bioterrorism. No wonder many call this dangerous step 'gunpoint medicine'.

Protests from various quarters – including high-profile political activists, public interest groups, the Association of American Physicians and Surgeons as well as average citizens – came to naught and both Acts have since been enshrined in law.

This despite shrill and loud public criticism, which pointed out that both acts gave governors and local bodies dictatorial powers and had considerable potential for misuse and abuse. Now here's a shocker. In November 2002, as if anticipating a 'pandemic', the US government included a rider in the Homeland Security Bill, which conferred immunity from liability prosecutions to vaccine manufacturers.

Why would a government, if not colluding with pharmaceutical companies, go to such lengths?

Terror had indeed cast a shadow longer than that intended by the alleged perpetrators of the September 11 attacks because the Patriot Act and MSEHPA, in one clear-cut swoop, potentially crushed civil liberties in the interests of preventing a "public health emergency". Was it a horrible overreaction by the federal authorities or is there more to this than meets the eye?

First, let us take a brief look at the background of the MSEHPA. The Act was commissioned to be drafted by the CDC and was drawn up by one of the CDC's attorneys Lawrence Gostin.

Gostin has been quoted in the *Journal of the American Medical Association* as advocating that with legal safeguards in place for citizens, "individuals should be required to yield some of their autonomy, liberty, or property to protect the health and security of the community".

Allow me to quote from the Act itself so that there is no ambiguity and so that you may read in black and white what US legislators, the people's representatives, have mandated. The MSEHPA states: *"During a public health emergency, state and local officials are authorized to use and appropriate property as necessary for the care, treatment and housing of patients, and to destroy contaminated facilities of materials.*

They are also empowered to provide care, testing and treatment and vaccination to persons who are ill or who have been exposed to a contagious disease, and to separate affected individuals from the population at large to interrupt disease transmission."

Yes, wily lawmakers can make even the most outrageous laws sound innocuous. Stripped of legalese and when translated into real terms, this is what it really means. The Act allows public health authorities to arrest (note the use of the term "separate") individuals, take away and burn their property and inject them with unknown substances (vaccines) if they were suspected to be carrying a contagious disease (even as simple as the common cold!). All this, as the Act claims, is for the "common good".

Suspending the Constitutional rights of 305 million people, the MSEHPA allows public health authorities to force American citizens to be vaccinated "with any medicaments selected by the State". Those who resist can be charged with misdemeanor, arrested and quarantined.

For those who think this is much ado about nothing and that no government would actually resort to measures as ridiculous as these, read on. The MSEHPA was initially drafted by Gostin immediately after the 2001 anthrax letter attacks soon after the September 11 terror assault. Typed up in less than a month, Gostin mentioned in his draft that he had prepared it in consultation with various national legal, legislative and health associations and bodies.

The author had to later retract this claim (lie) and drop it from later versions of the draft. If everything was aboveboard with the legislation (whose provisions suggest that this is clearly not the case), why did Gostin lie about a document as serious as this?

The final draft of this unconstitutional Act was released by the Centre for Law and the Public's Health. It is disturbing that since then, at least 39 states have passed bills after incorporating provisions of the MSEHPA.

1. WHO Decides Your Health?

What are the implications of forced vaccination? What happens when the government takes away your power to decide who can and who cannot inject toxic substances into you? What happens when the state controls your body?

This may sound alarmist but it is the sad truth – death has often resulted when decisions like this have been usurped from citizens. History is littered with medically documented cases where experimental vaccines have been administered under the guise of a 'public health emergency', with several fatalities.

What could be the government's possible motive? As discussed earlier (See Chapter 3: *Is There A Conspiracy?*), when governments, world health agencies and Big Pharma join forces, there are usually two broad objectives. The obvious reason is the billions of dollars that these lobbies and cartels gain from pushing toxic chemical doses on innocent citizens.

The second reason is an attempt to control weaker nations by, quite literally, further weakening them by, en masse, compromising the immune systems of the populace. A third reason cited by a group of people dubbed conspiracy theorists is an attempt at depopulation not unlike the grotesque eugenics experiments used by the Nazis during World War II.

Even when these motives are not present, sheer ignorance, callousness and lack of ethical considerations can cripple, maim and even kill babies and adults forced to get vaccinated with synthetic drugs, many of which have a dubious track record at best.

The Hepatitis B vaccine has long been associated with widespread and serious side effects. These include autoimmune diseases and neurological afflictions, including multiple sclerosis, arthritis, optic neuritis and lupus.

The Hepatitis B vaccine has also perhaps attracted more controversy than any other vaccine apart from being suspected to be the vehicle through which AIDS was 'introduced' into the human population. (See Chapter 3: *Is There A Conspiracy?*)

However, unmindful of these concerns, governments across the world have made the Hepatitis B vaccine mandatory for infants, and in some countries even prohibiting admission to kindergarten class if the child has not been vaccinated against the disease.

In France, however, after a prolonged battle and a public outcry, 15,000 citizens filed a class action suit against the government that resulted in the authorities halting the forced Hepatitis B vaccination campaign among school-going children. Unfortunately, the vaccine had already taken a heavy toll.

There are several global forums and alliances for mass immunization programs to ensure that control vests with a select group of influential people. While the public face of health is the World Health Organization (WHO), an interesting question to ask is who funds the WHO and its numerous programs that filter down to the millions of people who 'benefit' from them?

The fact is that some of the world's biggest philanthropic foundations and organizations as well as corporate houses sponsor some of the world's most notoriously controversial projects. And if you are wondering where all this is leading, you might want to bear just one thing in mind. These are the same individuals and groups behind WHO diktats on mass immunization and other so-called health programs.

Take, for instance, the Eugenics Movement, which started around the turn of the 19th century. The movement, in its present form, is a modern-day population control agenda spearheaded by wealthy developed nations concerned that a burgeoning 'third' world' is consuming large amounts of scarce resources that will deprive the 'first world' of these resources. Among these prized resources is oil.

Did you know that some of the most 'renowned' philanthropists such as John Rockefeller, Andrew Carnegie, Henry Ford and the Bill and Melinda Gates Foundation are among the frontrunners funding population control projects through mass sterilization programs and other measures in developing nations?

Did you also know that among the biggest donors of the WHO are the Rockefeller Foundation, Bill and Melinda Gates Foundation, Ford Foundation and Rothschild group of Britain? So we are faced with the question: Who controls WHO? And why?

During a recent TED conference presentation, Bill Gates answered this last question quite without hesitation and to the point. He said: "The world today has 6.8 billion people... that's headed up to about 9 billion. Now if we do a really great job on new vaccines, health care, reproductive health services, we could lower that by perhaps 10 or 15 percent."

Bill Gates has been a staunch advocate of population reduction for many years, and according to his recent statement he apparently knows how to achieve it. Mass vaccinations have repeatedly shown to cause progressively weakened reproductive health and infertility among vaccinated populations in Africa and Asia. If we do "a really great job on vaccines", we can certainly curtail the growth of these populations. In other words, these superwealthy individuals determine who and what country has a right to have children and who doesn't.

Vaccines that can destroy one's ability to have children are the ultimate weapon of controlling the future power balance in the world. Is this the true reason why these individuals and their foundations are so altruistic in their efforts to help rid the world of infectious diseases through their paid-for mass vaccination campaigns?

Is it really the desire of these "powers behind the scene" to help humanity survive by killing off a third or more so that the rest of us don't have to fight over the Earth's natural resources, or are they motivated by some even more sinister intentions?

These 'philanthropic' foundations work in the shadows; they influence legislation and exercise control over government policy through organizations such as the WHO, World Bank, UNICEF as well as governmental bodies such as the CDC and FDA. I don't believe they set up these and similar incredibly complex and influential organizations that are designed to assume the role of a world government just to make our life on earth easier. Those who control natural resources, food supply, water, travel and education control pretty much everything and everyone.

Add to this the nexus with Big Pharma and the picture fully unravels. When people like these exercise significant control over your health, they pretty much have control over your body, life expectancy, your children, and, in reverse, your ability to resist their methods and motives. Of course, it's a symbiotic relationship, with the world's biggest pharma companies funding these foundations and serving on their boards.

So the next time you stare at a vaccine vial, remember, it's probably not what it seems. But there is hope. There are enlightened citizens who have seen through these Machiavellian motives and who have stood up to mass immunization programs.

2. Forced Vaccinations

I will proceed to outline some cases of compulsory vaccination to show how governments conveniently trample on civil liberties and suspend constitutional rights to wrest control over the will of citizens.

Maryland: Remember the national anger when a court in Maryland (USA) dispatched summons to 1,600 parents in Price George's County, where children were not up to date on their vaccinations?

Following the court order, issued by the state Attorney General's Office in November 2007, parents and their children were herded into the court premises and forced to line up, in some cases, for as many as 17 doses of vaccination. Parents who refused to get their children vaccinated in court faced up to 30 days' jail time and a $50 fine for every day they "refused to cooperate".

The outrage was further fuelled by the double standards of the law enforcers: The state's attorney himself had refused to get his own children vaccinated against Hepatitis B, one of the most controversial vaccines available on the market.

This blatant violation of civil rights was provoked by a letter written by the school board, which had discovered that the medical records of more than 2,300 children did not comply with the state's requirements on immunization.

The manner in which the parents were literally forced, almost at gunpoint, to vaccinate their children, en masse, unashamedly violated the parents' right to informed consent. (This is somewhat similar to the Miranda Escobedo Rights of Silence read to individuals at the time of arrest.)

I say this because children cannot be vaccinated indiscriminately and prior to vaccination, doctors are bound to inquire into each child's medical history, previous vaccinations, inform parents about possible side effects and instruct them on how to monitor their children post-vaccination. This deliberate intimidation by the Maryland authorities is unconscionable.

Well, here's some more. The shocking truth about the Maryland forced vaccination drive is that it was motivated by cold cash. Some parents, who chose to scratch the surface, found that with 2,300 children being barred from attending school for failure to comply with mandatory immunization, the School District Board stood to lose funding from federal, state and other sources of up to $63 per child per day. Do the math and you arrive at a staggering sum. Obviously, the Maryland authorities – neither the school board nor the court nor the health authorities – had the children's health on their mind!

New Jersey: Maryland is not the only US state that had mandated compulsory vaccination for school children. A proposal drafted by New Jersey's Public Health Council took effect on January 1, 2009, making New Jersey the first state to mandate that toddlers who want to attend licensed pre-schools and daycare get vaccinated against the flu and pneumonia while children up to five years of age must get a meningitis and a booster DTaP shot.

Several months later, in August 2009, a US federal court issued an injunction that brought a halt to mandatory flu vaccinations in New Jersey and every other US state. According to the ruling, no citizen who refused to submit to flu shots should be denied any services or Constitutional rights.

Texas: With the federal authorities bringing vaccination under the purview of the Patriot Act, it seems constitutional rights are wide open to interpretation in the US. Taking the cue from the states of Maryland and New Jersey was Texas, whose Department of Health Services mandated additional vaccines for schoolchildren in April 2009.

The new schedule requires children seeking admission to seventh grade to take an additional meningitis shot and a tetanus shot that also ostensibly protects against whooping cough.

Children seeking admission to kindergarten will have to take a varicella vaccine shot if they haven't been administered the second dose of the two-shot vaccine, or if they haven't already had chickenpox. They will also need to be vaccinated against Hepatitis A and take two doses of the MMR vaccine.

According to the state Health Services, the enhanced vaccinations would "effectively eliminate the diseases in schools". Translated, this means 345,000 schoolchildren would receive massive amounts of foreign DNA, foreign RNA, fetal tissue and mercury that would effectively compromise their immune systems or leave them at risk for other diseases when they are older.

What happened in Texas was not unusual. Parents are usually 'hustled' into getting their children vaccinated before they are given a chance to explore the possible dangers of vaccination and before they can rally together to protest.

A barrage of emails and letters from the school and health authorities, vaccination 'camps' hurriedly organized on campus, and repeated coaxing from groups like the Houston Area Immunization Partnership predictably rushed parents into getting their children to line up to take the shots. The hustle and bustle left no room for parents to exercise their Right to Informed Consent, an issue I shall discuss later in this chapter.

Mothers in Peril: In October 2008, the National Center for Immunization and Respiratory Diseases, which is associated with the CDC, released yet another one of its many recommendations. This one was aimed at women who had just given birth. According to the recommendation, women in this category, as well as adolescent women of child-bearing age should receive the DTaP vaccine before contraception to reduce the risk of pertussis or whooping cough during pregnancy.

The DTaP vaccine is a chemical concoction that ostensibly protects against tetanus, diphtheria and pertussis, all of which can prove fatal to infants and adults with a compromised immune system. So far, the recommendation sounds just like one of the many routinely made by the CDC. But what was alarming was that a hospital in South Mississippi, Forrest General, was all but browbeating new mothers to get a DTaP shot before discharge from the medical facility.

I mention this as an example of how citizens' rights are once again usurped by healthcare agencies. This was not a case of forced vaccination but an example of how fear-mongering can coerce innocent people into saying "yes".

A woman who has just given birth is likely to be vulnerable and is more susceptible to manipulation. Hence, the likelihood of these women saying yes to the vaccine, especially when nurses and doctors say it is a recommendation of the CDC, is much greater.

Women in such situations must bear in mind that some hospitals, in an attempt to raise quick revenue, will act at the behest of drug companies and vaccine-makers, and will not think twice before potentially jeopardizing their patients' health. The point is that you must be vigilant and beware of vaccine pushers even in white coats!

Immigration Laws: Vaccine-makers are always on the lookout for captive populations. After all, it's a readymade market. While pushing its highly controversial Hepatitis B vaccine Gardasil, Merck & Co first targeted schools. It sparked a storm in Texas in 2007, when Governor Rick Perry (See Chapter 3: *Is There A Conspiracy?*) mandated that every female sixth-grader be vaccinated against the Human Papillomavirus Virus (HPV) with Gardasil to prevent cervical cancer.

Unmindful of the controversy, Merck & Co went ahead and recommended its vaccine to young boys for the prevention of genital warts. The FDA finally gave its approval for this purpose in October 2009 even as the vaccine maker had racked up billions of dollars in profits from the sale of this vaccine alone.

A year before that happened, Merck & Co took its sales pitch further with the US government, with the US Citizenship and Immigration Services (USCIS) making it mandatory for immigrants seeking legal permanent resident status in the US to be vaccinated against HPV.

This, unmindful of the serious concerns over the vaccine's track record, which has been associated with grave and even fatal reactions such as blood clots, strokes and Guillain-Barré Syndrome.

3. The Law On Forced Vaccination

If the law isn't confusing and sometimes even seemingly contradictory, the 2009 swine flu outbreak and mass hysteria whipped up during this 'pandemic' has further muddied the situation.

One state in particular – Massachusetts – has been in focus for its Pandemic Response Act that now allows the governor to declare a state of emergency and treat common citizens as terror suspects if they do not submit to forced vaccinations.

Despite the vociferous opposition from civil liberties groups, parents' forums, lawyers, consumer groups and other protesting concerned and enlightened citizens, the House of Representatives in August 2009 gave the bill a resounding thumbs-up.

Never before had any American state allowed the police to intervene in healthcare and vaccination. This legislation outrageously allows the police to forcefully enter people's homes without a warrant, forcefully quarantine residents, remove children from their homes and vaccinate them against their own will and that of their parents, and gives the state's governor the power to impose martial law. Of course, common citizens resisting any such attempts "in the interests of public health" can be jailed without charges or a trial.

As far as the law is concerned, when a state of pandemic is declared, citizens seem to have little choice but to submit to the State or face criminal charges. And the State, as it were, follows the diktats of the WHO, which has 194 signatories. This means that potentially, the populations of 194 countries could be subjected to measures such as those adopted in Massachusetts if their respective governments so choose!

These inexplicable measures – dubbed by many as 'Gestapo tactics' – have sparked a debate on what recourse citizens have when confronted by such tyranny. Many adults, parents and others have formed forums that take the anti-vaccination cause to their state's representatives in the hope that persuasive means will convince their political representatives not to use coercive tactics against the population.

However, it's an uphill task when you view mass vaccinations in a historical perspective. The law in favor of mass and forced vaccination dates back to the 19th century, when smallpox was rampant (See Chapter 2: Historical Blunders). This evoked a public backlash even then, with some states deciding to overturn these stringent laws.

The turn of the 19th century saw a landmark case that became the touchstone for all public health laws in the US – the Jacobson vs. Massachusetts case. In 1905, the US Supreme Court overturned a plea that forced vaccinations violated the right of every citizen to care for their own health. The court overturned the plaintiff's right in the interest of public health. The court had thus set the tone for state vaccination laws, and the Federal authorities have since vested with each state the power to make and enforce its own individual vaccination legislation.

However, the Supreme Court has always preferred to support the states in various lawsuits against forced vaccination, making the citizens' cause that much more difficult. Moreover, each state usually follows the guidelines of the federal authorities, which in turn follow the agenda of the CDC, which in turn is known to be partial to pharmaceutical companies. That's quite literally a vicious cycle.

The 1960s ushered in even more stringent legal controls, thanks to widespread measles outbreaks. After this, there was no looking back. Vaccine-makers were producing newer and newer vaccines and, ostensibly, vaccines against more and more diseases.

And there it was. Vaccine-makers had found a captive market for their toxic formulations – children. By whipping up fear in the minds of nervous and ill-informed parents, they along with policy-makers began to push their products through the school agenda, starting with playschool! It is no surprise that the number of vaccines mandated for babies and children has increased over the years.

Each state has its own vaccination laws with regard to what vaccines must be given and at what age and stage during a school-going child's life. And there's no escaping this public menace unless you choose to opt out of the system.

The fact is that parents who refuse to vaccinate their children are forced to withdraw their wards from schools. On the other hand, parents who do not send their children to school violate state truancy laws!

But there are certain rights every citizen possesses even in the face of forced vaccination. Indeed there are certain rules and regulations that public health authorities are bound to follow, again within the framework of the law.

Right To Informed Consent: No citizen can be forced to submit to vaccination. He or she must be informed of the possible risks, complications and side effects associated with the vaccine and other advisory material that the health authorities such as the CDC or FDA have made public. This information must be made available to the individual before any vaccine is administered.

The Right to Informed Consent is rooted in the National Childhood Vaccine Injury Act of 1986, which requires all doctors and other vaccine providers to provide parents written information about vaccines before their children are vaccinated.

It is this right that citizens and parents, in the case of mass school vaccination drives, are subtly deprived of. The scare-mongering, mass hysteria and psychologically coercive tactics adopted by the powers that be virtually frighten people into 'consenting' to being vaccinated. Under these circumstances, people are not likely to research a vaccine; they are more likely to take 'protective action'.

Exemptions: All 50 American states mandate a vaccination schedule for children seeking admission to various levels of school and college. Though the number and type of vaccines vary from one state to another, all state-licensed educational institutions have stringent vaccination rules.

But did you know that parents can refuse to submit to coercive diktats on medical grounds? For instance, if your child has a history of adverse reactions to earlier vaccination attempts, you may seek an exemption from further vaccination on medical grounds.

Different states have different requirements for applicants. While some states accept a simple written letter from a family physician detailing reasons for medical exemption, others reserve their right to review the recommendation and even override it.

The second ground on which an exemption can be obtained is religious as some faiths do not permit vaccination or any type of invasive medical treatment. While some states only broadly define the term 'religious beliefs', others require the applicant to be a member of a specific religious group of denomination. Again, while some require a letter of recommendation from the applicant's spiritual representative, others are more stringent and insist on an affidavit.

Exemption from vaccination based on religious grounds is rooted in the First Amendment of the US Constitution, which gives every citizen the right to freely exercise their religion. To take away this right and impose vaccination, the state must prove a "compelling state interest", which could be the spread of communicable diseases.

Interestingly, religious groups like the Amish who exercise this constitutional right don't permit vaccination in their communities and don't have communicable diseases and autistic children. This makes a lot of sense to me. I have never myself received a vaccine, thanks to my mother's great motherly, protective instincts. I have not seen a doctor in 38 years, given my healthy, strong immune system, and I have never had the flu in decades.

The third type of exemption is philosophical exemption, which constitutes an individual's personal beliefs that prevent him/her from being vaccinated.

This is the most subjective of the three types of exemptions but allow me to illustrate what happens when parents get together to mount a determined and organized effort to fight for their rights. It may have taken seven long years in Texas and two years in Arkansas but citizens in both these states finally won the legal right to exercise conscientious, philosophical or religious belief exemptions to vaccination.

Miffed by this hard-fought victory, state legislators are under increasing pressure from federal health authorities to revoke the exemption. As of 2010, 48 of 50 US states permit religious exemption while 18 allow a personal, philosophical or conscientious belief exemption from vaccination.

Of course, it is easier said than done as parents must comply with numerous formalities to seek an exemption, let alone be actually granted one. Not surprisingly, more and more citizens are resorting to this category to work their way around forced vaccinations. Not surprisingly, it has becoming increasingly difficult to secure exemptions on even medical and religious grounds.

Any which way you look at it, educating yourself on vaccination is the first step to preventing the state from invading your body. As mentioned earlier, all states have vaccination laws but they vary between states. Educate yourself on the laws pertaining to your state so that you can make an informed choice for you and your family. As more and more people are waking up to the harmful effects of conventional medicine, there are numerous forums and pressure groups which are rallying for the assertion of citizens' rights. Joining one of these forums might be a good idea.

Here is an example of what spending a few minutes on the Internet can reveal. For instance, a simple search will reveal that while the American Academy of Pediatrics and the CDC recommend that the MMR (measles, mumps, rubella) vaccine be given to all children, the law in your state may require children to be vaccinated against measles and rubella only.

Vaccination is becoming more and more pervasive in various aspects of life and may influence crucial choices and decisions in matters of adoption, child custody arrangements during divorce proceedings, eligibility for health insurance and government programs, medical care and immigration.

In a disturbing trend, which further illustrates the stranglehold of Big Pharma over the government and the medical fraternity, pediatricians have begun to refuse to offer medical treatment to children who have not fulfilled all vaccination requirements under the law.

There have been cases where hospitals have even reported parents to child social services agencies for their failure or refusal to get their child vaccinated. As outrageous as this may be, it's the bitter truth. Hence, it is more compelling than ever that you educate yourself on the law.

Soldiers: Army personnel, especially new recruits, are a favorite testing ground for vaccine-makers in mass immunization programs. Military troops have to submit to all manner of vaccinations in the name of readiness for warfare. Both men and women have little choice but to endure endless injections designed to 'protect' them against bio-toxins like smallpox, anthrax, ricin and other diseases.

Several soldiers have died from the often untested chemicals in these experimental vaccines, and others have been rendered severely sick by them. Not unlike women involved in involuntary ultrasound studies, soldiers have become guinea pigs in massive drug studies. How else could the pharmaceutical industry legally test poisons on human subjects?

Unfortunately, when you're in the armed forces, you have few civilian rights. Soldiers therefore do not have the right to refuse vaccination. Those who do refuse their shots face court martial and prison time, or at the very least, a dishonorable discharge.

Common side effects of the over one million vaccinations so far administered to US soldiers have included joint pain, extreme fatigue, and memory loss. The anthrax vaccine administered to Gulf War veterans in the 1992 war in the Middle East is one such instance. (See Chapter 3: Is There A Conspiracy?).

However, medical and religious exemptions are allowed but an exemption must be sought before enlisting. Once the recruit enlists with the armed forces, he/she pretty much signs over his/her body to the US Department of Defense which has been accused time and again of human experimentation.

4. Ever 'Herd' Of This?

There are several moral questions that arise out of forced vaccination – apart from the fact that is blatantly wrong. In this section, we shall discuss some of these nitty-gritty issues most people usually miss, thanks to the myths perpetrated by vaccine-makers in collusion with policy makers.

Now here is a question. If vaccines are indeed as effective as pharma companies make them out to be, why should we fear an epidemic or outbreak of a disease against which large sections of the population have already been vaccinated?

After all, vaccine-makers claim that vaccination offers 95 percent protection for a fully-vaccinated population. This implies that 5 percent of the vaccinated population has experienced vaccine failure.

In reality, this figure is way above the 5 percent failure that is implied though drug makers will never admit to it, at least not directly. During the rapid spread of a whooping cough outbreak in California in 2010, the health authorities urged the population to get revaccinated. Why would the population need to be revaccinated if they had already acquired immunity from the previous vaccination? Is twice-immunized better than once-immunized? Does this not imply that vaccines don't work? Hence the question: how can governments forcibly inject substances into the population when they know that there is a good chance that the drugs may not work?

There is another monumental fallacy used by vaccine-makers to push their agenda on an unsuspecting population: it's called 'herd immunity'. Flip the earlier statement about 95 percent immunity and this is how it reads: If 95 percent of the population is vaccinated against a disease, the population will be protected against it.

The problem with this argument is that it works with *natural* immunity, not artificially induced 'immunity'. This means that 95 percent of the population must be exposed to a disease, with some of them contracting the disease, for 95 percent to acquire natural immunity. Therefore, artificially immunizing the population will not offer the protection as promised.

As discussed in Chapter 1 on *The Vaccine Myth*, naturally acquired immunity indeed provides lifelong immunity while vaccines do not. Somewhere down the line, drug companies themselves discovered – and tried to cover up the fact – that vaccine-induced immunity (as measured by the mere presence of antibodies, which is not sufficient to protect against disease), often lasts about a decade, and sometimes for as little as two years, depending on the vaccine.

So they invented 'booster' vaccines, whose name implied that this toxic cocktail 'turbo-charged' the original vaccine. In reality, a booster is nothing but more of the same – another dose of the same vaccine. Hence, if you take a 'booster', you're actually being vaccinated against the same disease twice!

Next, another revelation for drug companies – boosters too didn't provide 'lifelong' immunity! Nature had checkmated even the most brilliant medical minds at their own game. So to cover up their own fallibility, vaccine manufacturers brainwashed the public into believing that a part of the vaccination schedule involves being vaccinated when you're an adult.

No wonder not just schools but colleges too mandate that applicants should take booster shots against certain diseases, even simple childhood diseases such as measles, chickenpox and mumps. Just like schools, collegians are another captive population that guarantees a ready market for vaccine-makers.

There is another implication of vaccine failure that puts paid to the arguments of the proponents of vaccination. If vaccines do not provide lifelong immunity and if the failure rate is significantly high, a large percentage of the population, especially those vaccinated around 50 years ago, must be walking around without the presumed protection!

Wouldn't that make at least half of America medically vulnerable to catching deadly contagious diseases? How is it then that we haven't experienced a massive epidemic in so long? We'll discuss why the swine flu outbreak of 2009 doesn't qualify for this argument in Chapter 7: *Swine Flu – The Pandemic That Didn't Pan Out.*

5. Scaring Up A Storm

It seems policy makers will never learn from mistakes of the past. That is often deliberate. I am referring to attempts to create 'epidemic' and 'pandemics', which are the biggest and most lucrative markets for vaccine-makers. Not only do pharma companies reap billions of dollars from the sale of their vaccines, but policy makers and senior public health officials also reel in massive kickbacks for awarding contracts for the manufacture of vaccines during these 'emergencies'. With the stakes so high, unleashing mass hysteria is the quickest way to make billions of dollars under a seemingly plausible pretext. Unfortunately, this usually has crippling consequences.

One such 'pandemic storm' hit the American public in 1976 during what has since been dubbed as the '1976 swine flu debacle'. Officially called the national Influenza Immunization Program, it was a disastrous mass vaccination campaign that is believed to have cost President Gerald Ford his Presidency and the Director of the CDC his job.

Three years later, in 1979, thanks to a scoop by the television station, CBS, the American public learnt the shocking truth behind the mass vaccination program. But by then, 46 million Americans had been administered the vaccine in question, 25 had died of it and

500 Americans were afflicted with Guillain-Barré Syndrome, a neurological disease that leaves victims paralyzed.

The debacle began in February 1976, when an Army recruit at Fort Dix in New Jersey took ill, collapsed and died at the army facility. A few days later, a handful of his colleagues exhibited the same symptoms but recovered. Next, two similar cases were reported in Virginia. Both individuals recovered. But this was enough to prompt the CDC to declare an outbreak of 'swine flu'.

The verdict of the CDC, which had processed throat cultures of the deceased army recruit as well as the others who later took ill was that they had all been infected with a 'swine flu-like' virus.

A month later, in March 1976, the heads of all public health agencies led by CDC Director Dr David Sencer virtually coerced President Ford to authorize a mass vaccination program across the US.

This campaign, which had the President famously declare that every "man, woman and child" should be immunized, cost the American tax-payers no less than $137 million, money that conveniently went into the coffers of pharmaceutical companies and doubtless of those in government who patronize them.

However, the program, which began in early October, was called off 10 weeks later after a severe public backlash. This was because within days of its launch, cases of Guillain-Barré Syndrome began to surface. It seemed, the vaccine had precipitated this rare neurological condition. By then, 25 percent of the American population had already been vaccinated.

But a deeper truth was yet to be revealed. In a 1979 interview to CBS, the television channel spoke to Dr Michael Hattwick who had directed the surveillance team for the swine flu mass vaccination program three years earlier.

In the interview, Dr Hattwick made a damning revelation: he had cautioned those spearheading the campaign that the vaccine carried the risk of neurological complications.

After first denying that Dr Hattwick had forewarned them but confronted with documentary evidence that the CDC was indeed aware of these consequences, Dr Sencer said that the "consensus of the scientific community was that the evidence relating neurological disorders to the influenza immunization was such that they did not feel that this association was a real one".

And thus so glibly did the CDC director, one of the so-called pillars of US public health, write the epitaph of at least 25 citizens and consign at least 500 others to a life of disability.

As a fallout of the disastrous 1976 debacle, the US federal government is still paying out billions of dollars in damages – again valuable tax dollars – to victims and their families who have since sued the government.

6. Pearls Before Swine Flu

If the government refuses to learn from mistakes of the past, history has taught many citizens valuable lessons. The swine flu outbreak of 2009 saw forced and mass vaccinations across the US and Europe but there is a growing tribe of enlightened citizens who are willing to stand up for their rights. The key to this heartening trend is educating oneself about the risks and dangers of vaccines and joining forces to put up combined resistance.

But before we discuss these encouraging examples, I'd like to focus attention on Germany and the public anger sparked by an announcement made during the swine flu 'pandemic'.

Amid the call for mass vaccinations in Germany, another controversy was playing itself out on the national stage. It seemed German Chancellor Angela Merkel, other politicians, military personnel, bureaucrats and the staff of the Paul Ehrlich Institute, an elite medical and vaccine research body, were superior to the rest of the population.

Public anger was sparked by the leak of an Interior Ministry document which revealed that it had ordered Baxter International's vaccine, Celvapan, for Merkel and the other elite while the rest of the population would receive Pandemrix made by GlaxoSmithKline.

The reason: Pandemrix contained an adjuvant called squalene, which has over the years been associated with serious neurological diseases such as multiple sclerosis, lupus and kidney disease as well as the notorious Gulf War Syndrome, among other equally debilitating consequences.

Celvapan, on the other hand, made by US pharmaceutical giant Baxter, did not contain the adjuvant and was associated with fewer side effects.

Setting the controversy at rest, a spokesperson for Merkel finally issued a public statement saying that should the German Chancellor get vaccinated, she would receive a jab of Pandemrix.

It is controversies such as these that confirm suspicions over the motives of governments, and the hypocrisy in the corridors of power betrays their complicity in committing crimes against humanity. Yet, compelled, as it were, they continue to follow a self-serving and crooked agenda, often with deadly consequences for the public.

But it is heartening that even as frightened citizens lined up at public health centers, and hospital emergency rooms and public places turned into temporary vaccination clinics and camps to get vaccinated against the swine flu en masse in 2009, protests were also brewing.

In Germany, newspapers reported an "open rebellion" by medical professionals and child physicians over use of the toxic vaccines for swine flu. In Denmark, healthcare workers and public officials refused to take the shot, saying the symptoms of the outbreak were mild and did not justify risking their lives.

A country-wide poll in Finland taken before the vaccine arrived suggested that 75 percent of the population would refuse to take the jab. A groundswell of resistance, if organized and focused on people's representatives, might just help overturn some of our draconian laws.

7. Flood Gates to Genocide?

Here is a question: What happens when you want to wash 'dirty money' and come off as a modern-day evangelist? Send it to the laundry. In this case, 'the laundry' is a multi-billion-dollar front for health programs that includes research on diseases and immunization experiments and campaigns conducted in developing countries.

And when you happen to be the richest man in the world, jetting around while projecting yourself as a savior comes easy. So while most of the world applauds software giant Microsoft founder Bill Gates for spending his fortune on fighting disease and devastation in developing countries, let us go behind this public relations exercise to discover the terrible truth.

It is ironic that Gates chose the following quote when announcing a $750 million initiative of the Bill and Melinda Gates Foundation, which by the way is America's largest foundation with an endowment of $24.2 billion from Microsoft Corp.

While launching the initiative, called the Global Fund For Children's Vaccines, Bill Gates had said in 2000: "It seems like every new corner we turn, the Rockefellers are already there, and in some cases, they have been there for a long, long time." Gates made that speech while announcing that his foundation was pledging $555 million to health programs across the globe.

I say ironic because the Rockefellers have been notorious in their funding of controversial research, dubbed by some as "genocidal". This research concerns depopulation programs, communist and socialist programs, 'mind control' or behavioral modification experiments and the notoriously controversial experiments of Alfred Kinsey.

But the Gates and Rockefellers are old friends and partners in the Global Alliance for Vaccines and Immunization (GAVI). The alliance, which controls major international vaccine programs, has the following as members: The Bill and Melinda Gates Foundation, the Rockefeller Foundation, the International Federation of Pharmaceutical Manufacturers Associations, UNICEF, World Bank, WHO and many national governments.

In vaccine research, it doesn't get bigger than this. I am detailing this to show just how incestuous the vaccine (and medical) world is. It also illustrates that power is concentrated in just a handful of entities.

As you continue to read this section, note how just one single foundation has neatly interlinked to various aspects of the vaccine agenda to a greater malady – perpetuating disease.

Is it any surprise that the Gates Foundation is using its immense clout in the debate on how to supply cheaper drugs for AIDS and other deadly diseases to poor nations? On occasion, the foundation has blatantly acted as a broker between developing nations and pharmaceutical companies.

This agenda of the foundation ties in nicely with another of its many global interests – promoting Anti-Retroviral (ARV) drugs in 'poor and AIDS-ridden' Africa. ARV drugs are on the cutting edge of AIDS treatment, and promoting these drugs props up the entire premise on which Big Pharma rests: that the drug cartel is a savior of the most dreaded disease known to man. The cartel therefore controls our health and even the health of entire nations, in this case, developing nations.

Here is another piece of the Gates Foundation pie. In 2008, the foundation announced 'Grand Challenges Explorations', a five-year $100-million initiative to scientists in 22 countries. The foundation said it wanted to "explore bold and largely unproven ways (read human experimentation) to improve global health".

How did it whitewash its image? Well, according to the foundation, it was aggressively promoting research into preventing or curing infectious diseases such as HIV/AIDS and finding a way around drug resistance (read ARV research).

In a media statement, the foundation had said something that may sound 'cutting-edge' to some but alarming when you read between the lines. It said the money was dedicated to projects that "fall outside current scientific paradigms". This massive infusion of funds went to universities, government agencies, non-profit organizations and six private companies.

Now let us take a look at just one reason why Bill and Melinda Gates would do the bidding of Big Pharma. In 2002, *The Wall Street Journal* reported that they had bought stock worth $205 million in nine major pharmaceutical companies, including Merck & Co, Pfizer Inc, Johnson & Johnson, Wyeth and Abbott Labs, manufacturers of anti-AIDS drugs and vaccines.

Soon after the news became public, eyebrows were raised over Gates's motives. Some suspect that his stock interests in pharma would further his intention to fight tooth and nail to protect the intellectual property rights of the big drug makers.

Concerns have arisen time and again over attempts by developing countries to seize patents so that they can produce affordable generic drugs for their populations. By taking the side of Big Pharma and thanks to his clout in developing countries, Gates can now almost ensure that patents remain with multinational drug companies and, consequently, that control over the health of weaker nations remains in the hands of a few.

Delve deeper and you realize that Microsoft in 2001 had named Merck Chief Executive Raymond Gilmartin to its board of directors. Gates and Gilmartin had worked together to launch a vaccine fund and the Microsoft founder had also helped Merck with an AIDS program in Botswana.

Yes, suddenly, philanthropy doesn't seem philanthropic anymore!

Chapter 5

The Vaccine Hangover

1. Vaccinating our children

Thirty-odd jabs in the first 18 months of life. That's how many times the average American infant gets vaccinated. Children in the United Kingdom are slightly better off. They get vaccinated only 25 times at this tender age.

And to make sure you're well and truly on the vaccination trail early enough, it is mandatory for babies to get nine or more different antigens pumped into their immature immune systems almost immediately after birth, some of them cocktails of more than one vaccine.

The best part for Big Pharma is that most of these vaccinations are backed by law. Children who are not vaccinated as per the CDC's schedule cannot enter or stay within the formal education system.

As if this arm-twisting were not enough, entire populations the world over are brainwashed into believing that they or their children will contract life-threatening diseases if they do not get vaccinated. And don't we all want the best for our children?

For many decades, leading scientists and doctors have vehemently promoted the idea that immunization of children is necessary to protect them from contracting diseases such as diphtheria, smallpox, polio, cholera, typhoid and malaria. Yet evidence is mounting, showing that immunization may not only be unnecessary but even harmful.

Pouring deadly chemicals into a lake doesn't make it immune to pollutants. Likewise, injecting the live poisons contained in vaccines into the bloodstream of children hardly gives future generations a chance to lead truly healthy lives.

'Willing' Victims

Children are most vulnerable because their immune systems are practically defenseless against the poisons in the vaccines. They have a lot going against them since their mothers do not pass on immunity through breast milk because *they* were vaccinated and no longer make certain antibodies.

The fact is that the human immune system has been designed to protect us from even deadly illnesses but the key here, as discussed in Chapter 1: *The Vaccine Myth*, is natural immunity. Vaccines, on the other hand, use synthetic chemicals to build artificial immunity. They work on the assumption that natural immunity is not good enough.

But could nature have made such a crucial mistake as to make us dependant on injecting foreign, toxic material into our blood when we have an immune system so complex and highly developed that millions of sophisticated computers could not imitate its performance? This is rather unlikely.

It is hard to believe then that these chemicals, which contain animal DNA, bits of weakened viruses, embalming fluid, mercury and other dangerous things are our modern-day life-savers. It is equally surprising that vaccines, which cause serious reactions and have debilitating effects on our health, are meant to stave off invading pathogens, many of which our bodies are designed to deal with naturally or are actually helping us to recover from a serious illness such as cancer. (For more details, see my book *Cancer is not a Disease – It's a Survival Mechanism*)

One of the main reasons vaccines are so dangerous is that they have never been tested for safety on human beings; they are only tested on animals. Vaccines cannot be proven safe until they are given to human beings for the first time.

But this would turn them into human 'guinea pigs' and it is not possible to predict what reactions they will have. This is the risk all people receiving vaccines have to take. Some will die, others will live but become ill years later, and many others will live without serious long-term consequences. But since all vaccines are designed to cause the very disease they are meant to prevent (to establish immunity), a truly safe vaccine is one that is not effective! Ironic, isn't it?

Under normal circumstances, all ingested foods, beverages, etc have to pass through the mucus membranes, the intestinal walls and the liver before they are permitted into such important areas as the blood, the heart and the brain.

The sudden appearance of a poison in the bloodstream is often met by a counterattack of the immune system that uses an entire arsenal of antibodies to heal the body from vaccine injuries and prevent death by poisoning. This is called an allergic reaction and in some cases, it could lead to a sudden, sometimes fatal, collapse known as anaphylactic shock.

Among the causes of anaphylactic shock are immunizations for (DTaP), Hepatitis B and whooping cough. A young person's immune system hasn't typically matured enough to withstand such an onslaught, resulting in what the medical fraternity calls Sudden Infant Death Syndrome or SIDS.

Noted researcher Dr Kenneth Bock points out that vaccinating children may make them hypersensitive to allergies, eczemas and certain foods, provoking acute reactions to a host of stimuli that are difficult to pinpoint. Vaccinations may therefore actually be sensitizing children to allergic disorders because the chemicals and genetic material in them change the way the immune system is meant to function. It becomes skewed with regard to the Th-2 hormone with a relative deficit in Th-1.

Some researchers go so far as to say that contracting some illnesses, such as mumps and measles during childhood, is healthy as they actually bring down the risk of allergies because they strengthen the immune system. The research I mentioned earlier clearly shows that the incidence of asthma and others allergy-related illnesses increases sharply following vaccination.

Fallacy & Fallout

Ever since Louis Pasteur proposed his erroneous germ theory of disease (See Chapter 1: *The Vaccine Myth*), the scientific establishment has linked a variety of bacteria, viruses and other pathogens to life-threatening illnesses against which pharmaceutical companies have devised an armor of protection in their little vials.

The problem is that despite their claims of success, certain vaccines have been consistently linked to specific symptoms and syndromes, some of which continue to baffle scientists and doctors even today. Among the various diseases that have been correlated to vaccines are chronic fatigue syndrome, autoimmune disorders, learning disabilities, encephalitis, growth inhibition, developmental disorders and hyperactivity.

Some of these issues, such as learning disabilities, were once dismissed as simple problems of growing up. Medical researchers now recognize them as forms of encephalitis (inflammatory disease of the brain). Here's a shocking statistic: More than 20 percent of American children – one out of five – suffer from these or related problems.

There is a mounting body of scientific research which shows that chronic diseases such as encephalitis, rheumatoid arthritis, multiple sclerosis, leukemia and other forms of cancer and even HIV may be provoked by vaccines administered in infancy.

For instance, rheumatoid arthritis, an inflammatory disease of the joints, was once an affliction of the elderly. Now, this crippling disease is widely prevalent among younger people and has been consistently associated with measles and rubella vaccinations.

Guillain-Barré Syndrome, a serious disease that leads to paralysis, is another syndrome which has been consistently associated with immunizations against measles, diphtheria, influenza, tetanus and the oral polio vaccine. This is hardly surprising when one considers the high toxicity of the vaccines. It is well-known that children whose immune systems are already weak experience more serious complications than those whose constitution and immune systems are much stronger.

Buying Into Myths

It is nearly impossible to estimate the damage and suffering that has been created and that will occur in future as a result of inadequate information about the dangers of modern immunization programs. Parents want to do what is best for their children and they carry a heavy burden of responsibility to keep them healthy and safe. Misinformation can create considerable conflict in parents because they don't want to neglect their children's health or cause them any harm.

Vaccine proponents argue that their chemical formulations have not just saved lives; they have also prevented epidemics and all but wiped out some deadly diseases from the face of the earth!

As discussed in Chapter 2: *Historical Blunders*, this is a myth. The truth is that the four leading childhood killer diseases – scarlet fever, pertussis or whooping cough, diphtheria and measles – had already declined by more than 90 percent before vaccines against these diseases were introduced! The reason these diseases vanished was that living conditions such as hygiene, sanitation and standards of living had improved significantly and people increasingly had access to healthy food.

This observation is supported by noted scholars who have researched vaccines such as Dr Andrew Weil. He points out that many serious diseases like cholera, typhoid, tetanus, diphtheria and whooping cough were on the decline in the last hundred years or so well *before* vaccines for them were even made.

Another reputed vaccine researcher, Viera Scheibner, points out that prior to 1940, the number of people perishing from diphtheria in Europe was negligible. But post-1940, when forced vaccinations were carried out on a mass scale against the disease, epidemics of diphtheria followed in individuals who had been fully vaccinated.

The 1940s also saw mass-scale immunization campaigns against whooping cough and tetanus across several countries. These too were followed by outbreaks of the so-called 'provocation poliomyelitis'.

Another problem with vaccination is that they are given indiscriminately, regardless of a child's health status. Many infants don't even get the chance to be healthy later in life because they are pumped full of these poisons against which they are helpless. At this stage of development, a baby has not yet acquired full natural immunity and has little ability to protect himself or herself.

The documented evidence against the value of immunization is so comprehensive that in 1986, the American Congress passed federal legislation to compensate children for damages arising from vaccination. According to the law, the government is no longer liable for damages but instead doctors and vaccine producers have to pay millions of dollars in compensation.

2. CFS: New-Age Polio

Chronic Fatigue Syndrome (CFS) or Chronic Fatigue and Immune Dysfunction Syndrome (CFIDS) is a condition associated with a constellation of symptoms that include a persistent, debilitating sense of tiredness or fatigue, muscle and joint aches and pains and symptoms of the flu like a sore throat, impaired memory and headaches and swollen lymph nodes. It is also referred to as Myalgic Encephalomyelitis or ME.

When triggered, the condition could last for months and even prevent some individuals from getting out of bed in the morning. It usually hampers normal functioning, prevents one from working and performing one's daily chores. It interferes with every aspect of life.

CFS, though very real to those who suffer from it, has been described as 'vague' because there is no obvious underlying pathophysiology associated with it. In other words, medical science is still unable to pinpoint a cause or find a remedy for this condition.

So what's the link between CFS and vaccines? The body of research on CFS suggests that the disease is consistently associated with infection, hormonal imbalances, decreased immunity and an abnormal reaction to infection. It appears to be a condition that can be triggered by many stimuli including vaccines. Let us discuss how vaccines can trigger CFS as a side effect.

Before we proceed, allow me to clarify what I mean by 'side effect'. I don't mean a temporary condition like a sniffle or a fever that goes away. While some symptoms may be temporary like soreness of the arm that is injected or a fever that lasts a couple of days, the side effects of vaccines are serious and persist throughout life.

These take place because the vaccine has fundamentally altered biochemical mechanisms in the body. These alternations, in turn, lead to structural and neurological changes that are serious and irreversible. In some instances, these consequences could even lead to death.

Researchers now believe that CFS can be set off by pathogens which trigger an abnormal immune response in the body. The human immune system consists of two types of responses – Th1 (T-cell Helper Type 1) response or cell-mediated immunity and Th2 (Th2 or T-cell Helper Type 2) response or the humoral response, where antibodies are primarily used to detect pathogens.

When pathogens enter the body, the immune system rings a 'Th2 warning'. It makes and releases antibodies into the bloodstream. These antibodies sense or recognize the pathogens as foreign, alien and potentially harmful agents.

Once this happens, the Th1 response kicks in. With the use of cells in the adenoids, tonsils, thymus, spleen, lymph nodes and lymphatic system, the immune system destroys, digests and ejects these pathogens, but not before the germs have helped the body to kill damaged, weak cells and decomposed toxins. This active attack constitutes what medicine calls the 'acute inflammatory response', which is associated with inflammation – fever, pain, malaise and the discharge of mucus or pus.

A healthy immune system uses both Th1 and Th2 responses to neutralize pathogens. Once the pathogen is destroyed and the attack subsides (read 'becomes unnecessary'), the immune system returns to its normal non-combat mode.

However, CFS victims exhibit an immune response that is skewed in two ways. One, they have a dominant Th2 response. Two, their bodies fail to switch off the Th2 response. As a result, the immune system is in a heightened state of combat even when not under attack. In other words, the immune system thinks it is fighting and protecting the body when, in reality, it doesn't have to, or so it seems.

In truth, the toxic ingredients of vaccines can severely impact liver functions and prevent the body from keeping itself toxin-free. In my book, *The Amazing Liver and Gallbladder Flush*, I describe how such powerful toxins can produce hundreds and thousands of intrahepatic gallstones that clog up the thousands of bile ducts in the liver which serve as the body's main detoxification routes. Consequently, vaccine toxins and other waste products that the liver is designed to remove end up in the delicate tissues of the organs and systems. This evokes an almost continuous immune response to heal the damage caused by the accumulated toxins and waste deposits.

This constant state of immune activation results in the chronic and debilitating sense of fatigue and other symptoms experienced in CFS. But it even if a causal link between the disease and its triggers still eludes science, it is possible to identify some situations and stimuli that set it off. One of these is vaccines.

There are a statistically significant number of cases where individuals who suffer from CFS had taken a vaccine just before its onset. A vaccine basically provokes the body's immune system just enough to create antibodies against a specific pathogen but not enough to provoke a full-blown inflammatory response. A vaccine is a way of artificially stimulating the body to respond in the same way it responds when it is detects a virus.

The answer to how and why vaccines evoke a CFS response is now fairly obvious: An immune system that leans towards the Th2 response (involving antibodies) and that does not switch off completely after it detects an infectious agent is provoked to react in the same way by a chemical vaccine.

Simply put, vaccines mimic the viruses that cause the disease they are designed to prevent; only, in milder doses. In CFS cases, the body cannot tell the difference between an infectious virus and a vaccine.

Some researchers have noted a link between CFS and specific vaccines, like the ones for Hepatitis B, cholera, influenza, tetanus and typhoid. The fact is that individuals who are prone to CFS, flibomyaliga, allergies and autoimmune disorders consistently report flare-ups after being exposed to various types of vaccines.

That's because all these conditions have one thing in common – an abnormal, heightened Th2 response.

Logically, these individuals should be forewarned about possible flare-ups if vaccinated. But do public health authorities ever educate the public about the possible risks? Do vaccines come with a contraindication for CFS patients? And with so many vaccinations being mandatory in the US (See Chapter 3: *Is There A Conspiracy?*), is it morally and ethically right for the government to force citizens to get immunized or be imprisoned as allowed by the Patriot Act?

What gives the government the right to play with human life, citing public health safety, and now, homeland security?

3. Polio by another name?

What if someone were to tell you that one of mankind's most dreaded diseases – polio – had not been eradicated as we have been led to believe? And that the medical fraternity is hiding a terrible, terrible secret?

Most people would greet a statement like this with a Pavlovian response that would go: "Conspiracy theorists." OK, let's start at the very beginning, rewinding to the 1950s and '60s, when the Salk and Sabine polio vaccines were introduced. The introduction of these two vaccines was indeed a medical milestone; only, not in quite the way most of us have been brought up to believe.

These vaccines certainly sounded the death knell of the three strains of polio virus which had allegedly killed millions of people around the globe before mass immunization against the disease was introduced.

The anti-polio vaccines, especially the oral polio vaccine developed by Albert Sabin, annihilated the polio virus that lives in the small intestine, on a mass scale. In doing so, the vaccine, administered to millions of people in forced vaccination drives around the world, had irrevocably altered the balance of nature in the human gut – it killed one type of virus and thus allowed others, kept in check by it, to proliferate.

These cousins of the polio virus – the Coxsackie viruses – also appear to damage the nervous system; only they do not cause paralysis that defines classic polio. After the polio virus was subdued, many of these other enteroviruses – 72 of them have been identified in the human intestine – began to cause polio-like symptoms on a widespread scale as they were allowed to proliferate and enter the bloodstream and brain.

This gave rise to a host of related neurological 'syndromes' (such a convenient term when the medical fraternity chooses to be confused) that began to show up with alarming regularity across populations. These include, hold your breath, CFS, Myalgic Encephalomyelitis, Multiple Sclerosis, Tourette's Syndrome, Guillain-Barré Syndrome, Idiopathic Epilepsy and, another favorite red-herring, 'Learning Disabilities'.

While polio damages the muscles, joints, heart, endocrine and lymph organs, these other syndromes lead to a greater variety of symptoms across the body. But it is more than pure coincidence that both CFS and polio have in common lesions in the brain stem, mid- and hind-brain and upper spinal cord. And this is just one of those 'pure coincidences'.

Hence, many researchers believe that these other syndromes are simply new forms of polio induced by the anti-polio vaccines, the price we have paid for tampering with nature.

4. MMR: Jaw-Dropping

Mumps: The MMR (measles, mumps, rubella) vaccine is among the most controversial vaccines. And a reminder of just why much of the 'eradication' hype is just hype comes from a wake-up call in 2009-2010 in the US.

The case I am referring to is an outbreak of mumps in more than 1,500 people in the states of New York and New Jersey in June 2009 and which spilled over well into 2010. The outbreak took place at a summer camp in New York and was traced to an 11-year-old boy who had just returned from the United Kingdom, where a mumps outbreak had spread to 4,000, mostly vaccinated, people.

Cases spread well beyond New York, to the neighboring state of New Jersey, as people returned home from the summer camp. But more than the outbreak itself is the fact that mumps is believed to have been eradicated in the US and that many of those who contracted the infection from the 11-year-old had been vaccinated against the disease.

This is what the Centers for Disease Control and Prevention (CDC) had to say in its report published in the February 12, 2010 edition of its Morbidity and Mortality Weekly Report.

"Most of the people who have become sick had received the mumps, measles and rubella vaccine (MMR). In fact, 88 percent had received at least one dose of the vaccine and 75 percent had received two doses."

But before you think the CDC had suddenly turned transparent and truthful, here's the 'disclaimer'. The report adds, "However, the vaccine is not 100 percent effective. Studies have found that one dose is 73 to 91 percent effective, while the effectiveness of two doses ranges from 79 to 95 percent."

I still cannot figure out the logic behind the CDC's argument. If, according to the CDC, the vaccine is not 100 percent effective, but rather 73-95 percent effective, how then is it possible that the vaccine failed to offer protection in the vast majority of the infected group (77 percent) that were fully vaccinated against mumps? The obvious question to be raised here is why does the unvaccinated population fare so much better in being healthy than the vaccinated population? Why should anyone get vaccinated against mumps when this so drastically raises one's likelihood of becoming infected with it?

The 11-year-old boy believed to have sparked the outbreak had also been 'fully vaccinated', which means he had received the two doses of the MMR vaccine mandated to make the vaccine 'effective'.

The CDC has also called the outbreak "the largest US mumps outbreak since 2006, when the US experienced a resurgence of mumps with 6,584 reported cases." This outbreak had taken place among college students. In this instance, most of the students who had contracted mumps had been 'fully vaccinated'. This is not surprising since a former head of the CDC said during the 2006 outbreak that "even when the vaccine is optimal, it is never 100 percent protective".

We are not asking for a 100 percent protection. A typical placebo-induced protection of perhaps 30-40 percent would be fantastic. But the mumps vaccine doesn't even get close to that. In fact, instead of protecting the population against mumps, the vaccine dramatically raises the people's chances of becoming infected with mumps.

Immunization against mumps is highly dubious. Even if it initially reduces the likelihood of becoming infected, the risk for mumps infection increases after acquired immunity subsides. In 1995, a study conducted by the UK's Public Health Laboratory Service and published in the Lancet showed that children given the MMR shot were three times more likely to suffer from convulsions than those children who didn't receive it. The study also found that the MMR vaccine increased by five times the number of children suffering a blood disorder.

126

In a report issued by German health authorities and published in a 1989 issue of the Lancet, the mumps vaccine was revealed to have caused 27 specific neurological reactions, including meningitis, febrile convulsions, encephalitis and epilepsy. A Yugoslavian study linked 1 per 1,000 cases of mumps encephalitis directly to the vaccine. The Pediatric Infectious Disease Journal in the US reported in 1989 that the rate varies from 1 in 405 to 1 in 7,000 shots for mumps.

Although mumps is generally a mild illness and the vaccine's side effects are severe, it is still included in the MMR vaccine. And so is the vaccine against rubella, although it is known to cause arthritis in up to 3 percent of children and in up to 20 percent of the adult women who have received it. It doesn't make any sense to vaccinate children against diseases that they can protect themselves from naturally.

In the case of mumps, for instance, children who get it in childhood remain immune to it permanently As Barbara Loe Fisher, President and co-founder of the National Vaccine Information Center, explains:

"Vaccines are supposed to fool your body's immune system into producing antibodies to resist viral and bacterial infection in the same way that actually having the disease usually produces immunity to future infection.

But vaccines atypically introduce into the human body lab-altered live viruses and killed bacteria along with chemicals, metals, drugs and other additives such as formaldehyde, aluminum, mercury, monosodium glutamate, sodium phosphate, phenoxyethanol, gelatin, sulfites, yeast protein, antibiotics as well as unknown amounts of RNA and DNA from animal and human cell tissue cultures.

Whereas natural recovery from many infectious diseases stimulates lifetime immunity, vaccines only provide temporary protection and most vaccines require 'booster' doses to extend vaccine-induced artificial immunity.

The fact that man-made vaccines cannot replicate the body's natural experience with the disease is one of the key points of contention between those who insist that mankind cannot live without mass use of multiple vaccines and those who believe that mankind's biological integrity will be severely compromised by their continued use."

Measles: Just like mumps, measles is not a dangerous childhood illness. The belief that measles can lead to blindness is a myth that finds it roots in an increased sensitivity to light during illness. This problem subsides when the room is dimmed and vanishes completely with recovery.

For a long time, measles was believed to increase the risk of a brain infection (encephalitis) which is known to occur only among children who live in economically backward localities and suffer from malnutrition. Among affluent children, only 1 out of 100,000 will become infected. Besides, less than half the children given a measles booster are protected against the disease.

Here is more evidence that vaccines do not work. The mortality rate from measles declined by 95 percent before the measles vaccine was introduced. In the UK, despite widespread vaccination among toddlers, cases of measles recently increased by nearly 25 percent.

The US has been suffering from a steadily increasing incidence of measles, although (or because) the measles vaccine has been in effect since 1957. After a few sudden drops and rises, cases of measles are now suddenly dropping again. The CDC acknowledges that this could be related to an overall decrease in the occurrence of measles in the Western Hemisphere. It had nothing to do with the vaccine.

In addition to this evidence, many studies show that the measles vaccine isn't effective. For example, as reported in a 1987 New England Journal of Medicine article, a 1986 outbreak of measles in Corpus Christi, Texas, found 99 percent of the victims had been vaccinated.

In 1987, 60 percent of measles cases occurred in children who had been properly vaccinated at the appropriate age. One year later, this figure rose to 80 percent.

MMR Vaccine: Apart from not protecting against measles and possibly even increasing the risk of contracting the disease, the MMR vaccine has been proven to produce numerous adverse effects. Among them are encephalitis, brain complications, convulsions, retardation of mental and physical growth, high fever, pneumonia, meningitis, aseptic meningitis, mumps, atypical measles, blood disorders such as thrombocytopenia, fatal shock, arthritis, SSPE, one-sided paralysis and death.

According to a study published in the Lancet in 1985, if children develop 'mild measles' as a result of receiving the vaccine, the accompanying underdeveloped rash may be responsible for causing degenerative diseases such as cancer later in life.

In 1994, the US Department of Health admitted to doctors that 11 percent of first-time recipients of the rubella vaccine would get arthritis. Symptoms range from mild aches to severe crippling. Other studies show a 30 percent chance of developing arthritis in direct response to the rubella vaccine.

Rather than pump a child full of chemical poisons engineered by human hands, it is far more prudent for parents to invest their time and efforts into building their children's natural immunity. Besides, allowing children to contract some of these childhood illnesses mentioned above may do more good than harm for their immune systems!

5. The HPV Hoax

The biggest side effect of the HPV vaccine is the fallacies being perpetrated by Big Pharma. For starters, how can vaccine maker Merck & Co claim that their vaccine Gardasil guards against 'the Human Papilloma Virus' (HPV) when this is a group of more than 100 viruses?

Misconceptions breed fear and then mass hysteria in the public. Put a price tag to that and you get a whopping $360 vaccine called Gardasil. Translate that into the millions of Americans alone who have been vaccinated with Gardasil and it's a staggering windfall for the pharmaceutical giant.

Let's do some digging for the truth behind the HPV vaccine, touted by the public health authorities as a savior for young women as it ostensibly protects against cervical cancer.

Here is how safe and effective this vaccine really is. As of September 2010, doctors across the US had clocked 65 deaths linked to Gardasil in reports to the CDC's Vaccine Adverse Events Reporting System (VAERS). Given the gross underreporting of adverse events to the CDC, this is a statistically significant number for a drug approved by the FDA in June 2006.

Apart from its damaging fallout, there are other problems with Gardasil (other than the fact that it is a vaccine!). It does not vaccinate against all types of carcinogenic HPV strains; its so-called protection lasts only a few years (See Chapter 3: *Is There A Conspiracy?*); and like all other vaccines, it is not foolproof.

Before we proceed, let us take a closer look at the vaccine and the HPV. Contrary to what public health propaganda leads us to believe, most women are infected with HPV at some point in their lives. Most of these women do not exhibit any symptoms and the infection subsides on its own in due course.

There are four types of HPV that are potentially harmful – the high-risk types 16 and 18, which are associated with 70 percent of cervical cancers; and the low-risk types 6 and 11, which are associated with lesions or warts in the throat and genital tract. These are sometimes considered pre-cancerous.

Gardasil contains bits of all four types of virus, material that has been genetically modified. However, this much-publicized vaccine has kicked up a storm ever since it was approved by the FDA. It first raised eyebrows when the FDA fast-tracked it for clearance. All this fuss over a disease that accounts for only 1 percent of cancer deaths in the US!

But the stakes were high – its price tag – and it was no surprise that the government seemed more concerned than the public that the HPV vaccine should be out on the market at the earliest. But here's the real coup, a bitter irony. In January 2010, the pharma giant announced that the Director of the CDC from 2002 to 2009, Dr Julie Gerberding, had been appointed President of Merck Vaccines. Finally, all that Gardasil-pushing made perfect sense!

How Adverse Is Adverse?

According to the non-profit organization Judicial Watch, Gardasil was associated with around 9,000 'adverse events' in the first two years after it was approved. These included 18 deaths. Post January 2008, 140 'serious' events have been reported, 27 of them 'life-threatening', in addition to 10 spontaneous abortions and six cases of Guillain-Barré Syndrome (GBS).

Further research revealed that there were 38 cases of GBS logged with the FDA since June 2006, including the six mentioned above. GBS is an autoimmune syndrome where the immune system attacks the body's own nervous system (or rather the toxins accumulated there), often leading to paralysis and in some cases, death. GBS, as mentioned earlier in this book, is one of those diseases like allergies that have seen a dramatic rise in the post-vaccination era.

There is more. Classified documents procured from the FDA under the Freedom of Information Act revealed that some of the women who had been vaccinated with Gardasil experienced sudden blisters on the back and arms, warts in the genital area, vaginal blisters within just two days of being vaccinated and these blisters then spread to other areas of the body.

Upset with these revelations, the FDA and Merck called these symptoms a "coincidence" and stated that the VAERS reports did not establish a cause-effect link between Gardasil and the symptoms. Alternatively, one may wonder why doctors, nurses and patients would take the trouble to file reports with VAERS if they thought the symptoms were not connected or serious enough to report. How can the FDA and Merck make such subjective statements and declare them to be the truth, if they have no proof to substantiate their claims. Are 18,000 "coincidences" not enough to at least wonder whether there is a connection between Gardasil vaccinations and these reported side effects?

Many researchers point out that there have been a significant number of cases where genital and other warts have broken out immediately after the vaccine was administered to young women. Like with other vaccines, Gardasil had triggered the very disease it was meant to guard against. An infection caused by a vaccine is far more likely and logical than a coincidental occurrence of such side effects.

But ethics is the forte of neither Big Pharma nor public health authorities nor lawmakers. That is why Merck spent millions of dollars marketing its 'wonder drug' in two ways, both of which invited such a strong public backlash that the vaccine maker had to withdraw its campaign.

One, Merck began its hardsell well before Gardasil was even approved by the FDA. It virtually blitzed the drug on television and the Internet in an attempt to scare up a storm so that young women would make a beeline for the vaccine once it was on the market.

Second, Merck spent millions of dollars lobbying with state and federal authorities and lawmakers to make Gardasil mandatory for schoolchildren and even preschoolers. It almost succeeded! (See Chapter 3: Is There A Conspiracy?) Many states went so far as to draft legislation to make the vaccination mandatory in school but due to public outrage and vociferous consumer groups, Merck suspended its lobbying campaign in 2007.

How Dire Is Dire?

There is another reason the marketing campaign mounted by Merck rings hollow. Again, let us return to pure statistics to see just how dire it is to have a vaccine against HPV. According to data with the American Cancer Society, the incidence of cervical cancer in the US plunged more than 70 percent between the 1950s and 1990s.

Here is another statistic. Cervical cancer is not even listed in the top 10 cancers in the US. Among those with the highest prevalence are lung, breast and colon cancer. So why was the FDA fast-tracking a drug and why were lawmakers so anxious to pass legislation making Gardasil vaccination mandatory for a cancer that keeps declining and was far from even ringing alarm bells in the population?

The drug giant was clearly not interested in helping out a handful of young women who may have been at risk of developing cervical cancer later in their lives. Rather, it wanted to open up a huge potential market for cancer vaccines.

Merck's own literature says it is important to realize that Gardasil does not protect women against some "non-vaccine" HPV types. In other words, even if girls accept the risks and get vaccinated, they can still get HPV!

Blood Money

But could there be another reason why Merck went into overdrive over Gardasil? Rewind a few years to the scathing controversy and subsequent recall of Vioxx, a pain-reliever made and marketed by Merck for arthritis patients.

The drug was recalled in 2004 after damning testimony from the FDA's Office of Drug Safety (ODS) during Senate hearings. In his testimony, Dr David Graham, associate director for science and medicine with the ODS, admitted that Vioxx had caused an estimated 38,000 heart attacks and sudden cardiac deaths.

Graham also said this was a "conservative estimate" and that the number of heart attacks could be anywhere between 88,000 and 139,000, of which "30-40 percent of the victims had probably died".

Five years later, the ghost of Vioxx reared its ugly head for Merck. In November 2009, court proceedings in a case where the drug company was being sued over Vioxx brought out classified data that Merck had kept concealed. The data revealed that the company had known about Vioxx's 'killer effect' for three years before it came to the public's attention. In other words, the drug makers knowingly and willingly let elderly arthritic people die of a drug it had made simply to protect its reputation and safeguard profits.

Interestingly, as the shocking truth about Vioxx tumbled out of Merck's closet, the company was already cooking up its next scam –

Gardasil. So just as the company suffered a blow that could have destroyed the drug maker, it was already making a vaccine that it hoped would both salvage its reputation and rake in some of the billions it was losing in lost sales and Vioxx lawsuits. But who said drug companies had a conscience?

6. Hepatitis B: Baby Killer

The Hepatitis B shot is one of the first vaccines newborns receive. Yet there are no benefits to the baby. This is because the medium through which the Hepatitis B virus spreads is blood and blood products, and infected needles, intravenous drug use and unprotected sexual contact.

So unless a baby is a junkie or is engaging in dangerous sexual practices, there is absolutely no benefit (even as far the dubious benefits of vaccinations go) to a baby receiving the Hepatitis B vaccine.

Moreover, even vaccine manufacturers admit that the alleged efficacy of the Hepatitis B vaccine wears off within seven to ten years, and even faster in children. Hence, even for those who accept that vaccination is beneficial, what justification could there be to mandate a vaccine for a section of the population that receives absolutely no benefits from it?

This is why. The Hepatitis B vaccine was commercially introduced in 1986. It was essentially a vaccine that was meant to protect against a disease prevalent among select, high-risk groups of the population as the Hepatitis B virus spreads only through blood, blood products and body fluids. These high-risk groups included drug users, homosexuals and those engaging in unprotected sex.

The problem is that these high-risk groups, who are most likely to contract the virus, are also least likely to get vaccinated. So Merck, who manufactures and markets the vaccine in the US, needed to look for new markets. Quickly.

Five years after the Hepatitis B vaccine hit the market, in 1991, the CDC did a sudden about-turn, one that opened up a whole new market for the vaccine maker. And the agency came up with some remarkable jugglery.

Not surprisingly, it was the same agency which had, before that, taken pride in announcing that the US was among the countries with the lowest incidence of Hepatitis B (0.1–0.5 percent of the population) – just 18,000 cases in a population of over 240 million.

At the end of 1991, the CDC's Advisory Committee on Immunization Practices (ACIP), no doubt at the behest of Merck, suddenly recommended that all infants be administered the first of three doses of the vaccine within a maximum 12 hours of birth!

Next, the CDC threw up some unbelievable figures to justify this recommendation, estimating that the US had around 1.25 million people with chronic Hepatitis B infections. The agency said that about 4,000 to 5,000 of these people die from chronic liver diseases annually. For good measure, it added that in the decade before its recommendation, 200,000 to 300,000 new Hepatitis B cases were detected every year!

Hence, by allegedly winning over government officials and policy makers with financial incentives, Merck was able to get governments in developed countries to make the Hepatitis B vaccine mandatory at birth. At $50 for the three-dose vaccine, the pharmaceutical company was now raking in at least $1 billion in sales from this vaccine alone every year.

In the process, it was able to get the vaccine administered to millions of babies who would receive no benefits from this toxic cocktail, and whose immune systems would, in fact, be compromised *because* of it.

The government's chicanery was so powerful that it got the public to ignore another set of figures that would have bared the truth about just how 'dire' the need for the vaccine was. The fact is that about half the number of individuals who do contract the illness exhibit no symptoms of the disease while also acquiring permanent immunity from it. Another 30 percent individuals who contract the virus experience flu-like symptoms while only the remaining 20 percent actually exhibit symptoms. Of these, *a further 95 percent* recover completely.

This means that only 5 percent of individuals infected with the Hepatitis B virus become chronic carriers. Now get this. Of this group, only a quarter, or 25 percent, suffer from chronic liver disease or cancer. That's a statistical minority – 1.25 percent of the number of individuals exposed to the virus – who are at serious risk. How does this make the Hepatitis B virus a threat to public health? How does this justify mass vaccination? Why not allow people to voluntarily choose to take the vaccine?

Numbers Don't Lie

But why exactly is the Hepatitis B vaccine so dangerous? The last place you will find an answer to this baffling question is the CDC and FDA's VAERS system. According to VAERS's public records, there were only 19 cases of infant deaths linked to the Hepatitis B vaccine reported in the last decade of the 20th century.

However, according to one independent researcher, who obtained raw VAERS data not normally in the public domain, there were actually 54 reports of infant deaths relating to the Hepatitis B vaccine between January 1996 and May 1997 alone. None of this was made public through VAERS! And these were only cases reported by doctors, nurses, parents, etc to VAERS.

The researcher also learnt that reports of 17,000 adverse reactions to the vaccine had been logged by VAERS during this period but none of these had been made public by the FDA and CDC.

When the Hepatitis B vaccine was introduced, it was touted as the safest way to guard against a virus that could cause irreparable damage to the liver, lead to cancer and eventual death. Its introduction as a mandatory vaccine and the mass immunization campaigns in the US in the late 1980s and 1990s were highly controversial also because of the suspicion that this vaccine had been used by the public health authorities and US government as a vehicle to introduce the HIV virus to select groups of the American population. (See Chapter 3: *Is There A Conspiracy?*).

As researchers dug deeper, more skeletons began to tumble out of classified government and military closets, much to the public's horror. Yet the US government and policy makers had succeeded in making this vaccine mandatory for infants across the population.

However, the French government was forced to respond to public concerns, especially after thousands of French citizens sued the government for concealing the risks associated with this vaccine. After its introduction in France, hundreds of people reported autoimmune and neurological symptoms and other demyelinating diseases, which included multiple sclerosis. The Hepatitis B vaccine was thus pulled off the list of vaccines mandated for school children by the French government in October 1998.

Autoimmune Link

The Hepatitis B vaccine has been the subject of intense research as well as debate due to the vaccine's association with 'new-age' autoimmune disorders. These concerns have arisen due to vaccine-induced reports linked to developmental disorders, attention deficit disorders, learning disabilities, autism, encephalopathies that cause permanent brain damage, Chronic Fatigue Syndrome, multiple sclerosis, rheumatoid arthritis, asthma and seizures.

Research also suggests that the earlier the age of vaccination with the Hepatitis B vaccine, the greater the likelihood of developing insulin-dependent diabetes, which is also an autoimmune disorder.

This disturbing correlation can be explained by the fact that vaccines, including the three-dose Hepatitis B vaccine, overwhelm the developing immune system of a newborn baby. In fact, the immune system of an infant does not react in the same way to pathogens and antigens as does the adult immune system.

So why doesn't everyone who receives the Hepatitis B vaccine fall sick? According to researchers, the vaccine, which uses recombinant genetic material, mimics human proteins in a way that confuses the human immune system. As a result of this mix-up, the immune system mistakes the body's cells for foreign pathogens and starts attacking its own cells and tissues. This is the basis of an autoimmune disease.

There is a statistically significant percentage of the population that is prone to this 'cellular confusion', individuals whose genetic tendency to be confused once the vaccine enters the bloodstream experience flare-ups or full-blown neurological and other symptoms characteristic of autoimmune disorders.

However, when people are vaccinated, it is important to be aware of the risks involved. These vary between vaccines and between individuals. How would you know if you're predisposed to an autoimmune disorder if you haven't experienced symptoms and therefore been tested before? Should you get a genetic profile performed prior to being vaccinated? Do the packet inserts that come with vaccines tell you the whole truth about these chemicals? Do you even need to be vaccinated?

Concerns over the safety of vaccines have been growing in recent years, thanks to the spread of information over the Internet. With so much information out there, it is hard to hide the lies. So if vaccine packet inserts are ambiguous and incomplete, the public doesn't depend on the fine print and family physicians for information any more.

Parents in the US are increasingly questioning the need to have their children receive as many 30-odd vaccines by the age of 18 months. So to cloak the number of vaccines and downplay the assault on the babies' immune system, vaccine manufacturers resort to another ploy.

They combine vaccines into a single shot, or vaccine cocktail, as is the case with the DPT (diphtheria, pertussis and tetanus) the MMR vaccine (measles, mumps and rubella) and the MMRV vaccine (measles, mumps, rubella and varicella for chickenpox)!

Now here's disturbing news for parents choosing to get their children vaccinated with a combination vaccine – one that combines the MMR and chickenpox vaccines. The Kaiser Permanente Vaccine Study Center, which used the government's Vaccine Safety Datalink, found that children who receive the combined vaccine are almost twice as likely to develop fever that leads to convulsions than those who don't.

According to the study, whose results were published in the journal Paediatrics in July 2010, the risk of febrile convulsions was observed to be 1 in every 1,000 children who receive the MMR vaccine and increase significantly when toddlers receive the MMRV vaccine. The researchers concluded: "Vaccination with MMRV results in 1 additional febrile seizure for every 2300 doses given instead of separate MMR + varicella vaccines.

It is a matter of increasing concern that governments, public health authorities and policy makers have given Big Pharma the go-ahead to raise generation upon generation of immuno-compromised children. This in a day and age when pollution levels are at their highest, lifestyles are encouraging disease, and processed and genetically modified food is weakening and even altering (for instance in the case of obesity) human metabolism. It's a sad irony that we are weakening, rather than strengthening, our children who are faced with health hazards like never before.

It was therefore heartening, albeit surprising, to see a Fact Sheet released by the World Health Organization (WHO) cautioning against corruption in the pharmaceutical business. The Fact Sheet points out that corruption takes place at all levels and at every step of the process – from research and development, to developing a drug or vaccine, to securing approvals and licenses, to advertising and marketing drugs, to what drugs are listed in which health program, to drug regulation by government health agencies.

The WHO admits that as much as $12 billion to $23 billion of health care spending is lost to unethical practices and other types of corruption in developed countries every year. Apart from the comment on pharmaceutical companies, the alarming part is what the public is faced with once a drug or vaccine trickles down the supply chain.

There is no way of telling what many vaccines actually contain, what consequences they may have and whether many of these drugs should even be on the market. Drug scandals and repeated drug recalls are a testament to the risk that vaccines pose to our health rather than the protection they pretend to offer.

The Rotarix Scandal

But how do you explain this scandal to the parents of 30 million children around the world, including 1 million in the US? This is the number of children who were vaccinated with Rotarix, a vaccine made by GlaxoSmithKline and approved for use in the US in 2008, to ostensibly protect against the rotavirus, an organism that leads to severe diarrhea in children. Rotarix is typically given to infants at two and four months of age.

According to the FDA, preliminary results from a study in Mexico involving GlaxoSmithKline Rotarix vaccine suggest an increased risk of a serious bowel problem that could be fatal. The announcement appeared in The Wall Street Journal on September 22, 2010. This study clearly proves that vaccines can produce the diseases they are supposed to prevent, or worse.

A statement posted to the FDA's website said the study showed an increased risk of intussusception in the 31-day period following the first dose of Rotarix. Intussusception is a twisting or obstruction of the intestine that can be fatal. Of course, the FDA has no intention of pulling the dangerous vaccine off the market, although this vaccine has had a history of being a trouble maker.

Licensed in 2008, Rotarix was temporarily pulled off the market by the FDA in March 2010 after the discovery that the vaccine was contaminated with a pig virus (porcine circovirus PCV1). It is a foregone conclusion that all 30 million children who received this vaccine also received the pig virus because the seed stock, or the original cell bank from which all the vaccine doses were subsequently created, was contaminated with this swine virus.

The contamination was discovered by a team of researchers who were studying the purity of vaccines made from live attenuated (weakened) viruses. The list included the vaccines for rubella, polio, chickenpox, yellow fever, measles, MMR and rotavirus.

- What they found was shocking:
- Porcine circovirus PCV1 in Rotarix
- DNA fragments from the avian leukosis virus in the measles vaccine
- DNA fragments of a virus similar to a simian retrovirus in RotaTeq made by Merck

It is not unusual for fragments of animal genetic material or DNA to be found in vaccines. It is the type of material that could prove lethal. Viral material is obviously one of them. Remember the stunning SV40 discovery in the live polio vaccine? (See Chapter 2: Historical Blunders)

So, how did PCV1 find its way into the Retorix vials? In addition to other animal tissues and serum (monkey and cow) used to develop the Rotarix seed stock, porcine trypsin, an enzyme in the pancreatic juice of pigs, was also used in its manufacture. PCV1 had entered the seed stock while adding the porcine trypsin to the stock. But since when have vaccine-makers been checking? They certainly don't intend to commit financial suicide. If every vaccine they produce were to be checked for contaminants, the vaccines would never sell.

7. DPT: Sudden Death

Fear is one of the most effective weapons used by vaccine-makers to get parents to submit to the 'dangers' of disease while offering a panacea for their children. It doesn't matter to vaccine-makers that their 'persuasive' tactics cause the deaths of scores of babies every year.

I am referring to the DPT (diphtheria, pertussis, tetanus) vaccine, which has been implicated time and again in cases of Sudden Infant Death Syndrome or SIDS. (See Chapter 3: *Is There A Conspiracy – War On Infants*).

Research confirms that the pertussis or whooping cough vaccine is only effective in 36 percent of children. A report by Professor Gordon Stewart, which was published in 1994 in *World Medicine*, demonstrated that the risks of the whooping cough vaccine outweighed its benefits.

DPT, the whooping cough vaccine that was used in the US till 1992, contained the carcinogen formaldehyde, and the highly toxic metals aluminum and mercury. Both this vaccine and its 'improved' version, DTaP, have never been tested for safety, only for 'efficacy'.

The new vaccine has proved to be no better than the old one. Both versions cause death, near-death, seizures, developmental delays and, at the very least, hospitalization. DTaP is given to babies as young as six weeks old although the vaccine has never been tested on this age group.

Another reminder of the dangers of the DPT vaccine came in July 2010, during an outbreak of whooping cough in California where 10 infants died of the illness and nearly 6,000 cases were confirmed to this day (November 1, 2010). In fact, public health authorities have admitted that there has been a resurgence in pertussis in recent years, with a sudden rise in the disease every now and then. This despite (or because of?) the fact that the vaccination rate of DPT being very high.

In the wake of the outbreak, the CDC admitted that the pathogen may have adapted to the vaccine, a fact supported by the observation that Bordetella parapertussis, a relative of the Bordetella pertussis bacteria which causes whooping cough, can also cause the disease in immune-deficient individuals, especially in young children. Some researchers suspect that the DPT vaccine may have weakened the immune system (the vaccine contains large amounts of bioactive toxins) so much that it left victims vulnerable to attacks from the Bordetella parapertussis bacteria.

All vaccines damage the immune system and this makes infants especially vulnerable to bacterial infection. Since there is no real safety testing done on vaccines, vaccine-makers and doctors cannot be directly blamed for causing such epidemic outbreaks. In fact, just the opposite happens: health officials blame the lack of vaccination among infants and adults for the outbreak, scrambling to educate and inform people about the importance of vaccination.

According to Dr. Jennifer Ashton, CBS News' medical correspondent, since it is not possible to vaccinate infants under two months of age, it is extremely essential for adults living and working with children to get vaccinated, or revaccinated.

Yet, there is no proof that the pertussis vaccine prevents whooping cough. Someone is just making this up. It is just as likely that vaccinated adults spread the illness to their already immune-compromised children. According to statistical evidence, numerous epidemics started immediately after immunization programs were introduced to the population. Why should this latest outbreak make an exception to this rule?

The infection starts out like the common cold in adults and children, with mild coughing and runny noses. Typically, it takes a week or two for the violent cough that sounds like a harsh bark to make an appearance, though some cases of pertussis do not produce the characteristic cough.

The overuse of vaccines is a risky endeavor. Just as overuse of antibiotics has lead us to the onset of deadly antibiotic-resistant organisms (superbugs that cannot be destroyed), constantly inoculating the population with pathogen-filled vaccines can cause the pathogens to adapt to the vaccines and render them useless (according to the CDC's own admission).

Returning to our discussion on SIDS, among the 17 potential health problems caused by the whooping cough vaccine, SIDS tops the list. According to an estimate from the University of California at Los Angeles, 1,000 US infants die every year as a direct result of receiving the vaccine. Children die at a rate that is eight times faster than normal after a DPT shot. James R Shannon of the National Institutes of Health understood this when he said, "No vaccination can be proven safe before it is given to children."

Health authorities claimed that the 10 deaths which occurred during the recent outbreak in California were due to the fact that these infants were not vaccinated. This is highly unlikely since the vaccine is only effective in 36 percent of children; accordingly, 6 or 7 children would have died anyway. Besides, there may have been other serious pre-existing health conditions that could have contributed to their death, which so often is the case when a typically non-lethal infection such as pertussis kills someone.

While it is a great tragedy for any parent to see their child die just weeks after it was born, it doesn't even get close to the tragedy of the 1,000 children who die unnecessarily each year as result of being vaccinated against whooping cough. It is difficult to understand how any doctor, health official, or drug company CEO can stand up with a clear conscience and announce that it is perfectly okay to let 1,000 children die in order to save 10 other children. Or are they just ignorant about the truly important published research and instead blindly trust in myths and pseudoscience? Or are they just greedy and don't care?

Also, diphtheria is still combated with toxic immunization programs even though it has almost completely disappeared from the planet. When diphtheria broke out in Chicago in 1969, 11 of the 16 victims were individuals who had been immunized against diphtheria. In another report, 14 of the 23 victims were completely 'immune'. This shows that vaccination makes no difference when it comes to protection against diphtheria; on the contrary, it can even *increase* the chance of being infected.

Mini-Strokes

Researcher Dr Andrew Moulden, an expert in neurobehavioral assessment of brain and behavioral disorders, has made some interesting observations about vaccines after years of extensive research. He says vaccines, across the board, cause ischemia – restricted or impaired blood flow in microcirculation units. This is a level that is so microscopic that it is difficult to observe.

According to Dr Moulden, vaccines lead to ischemia, which in turn leads to anoxia or impaired oxygen delivery to tissues. This, in turn, leads to cell death or mini-strokes. When this takes place in the brain and nervous system, it leads to neurodevelopmental disorders such as CFS and learning disabilities. It could also take place in cells and tissues elsewhere in the body. This is how vaccines produce a variety of symptoms, depending on the damaged area.

Dr Moulden says that when a vaccine is injected into the blood, two things take place. One is non-specific immune hyperstimulation or immune hypersensitivity. The second is an electrostatic instability of blood flow that impairs fluid dynamics and oxygen/nutrient delivery throughout the body's vascular system. Healthy blood flow is the basis of life, healing, cellular function, wellness and health, he points out.

Dr Moulden explains that one of the processes that takes place is the waxing and waning, and acute, then chronic, changes in blood flow from 'fluid to 'gel'. For instance, aluminum present in vaccines as an adjuvant causes 'sludging' of blood flow. This takes place as aluminum causes particles in the blood to agglomerate, giving the blood a sludge-like quality.

The capillaries cannot absorb oxygen and nutrients from 'thickened' blood, which leads to cellular and tissue damage. If this seems 'minor', it is not when taking place at the microscopic level, explains Dr Moulden. He says infants who die suddenly and 'inexplicably' after being vaccinated suffer impaired blood flow to end-capillary vessels in the brain stem, which controls the reflex-like respiratory response.

All individuals who are vaccinated thus suffer a series of ischemic strokes throughout life. When the body reaches 'breaking point', it results in neurodevelopmental and other disorders, explains Dr Moulden.

Medical science has miles to go before the adverse effects of vaccines are fully understood. Suffice to say that a healthy immune system and an overall healthy lifestyle is the best protection against disease.

Chapter 6

Autism: Mercury Assault

If you turn back the clock, history will show you that the origin of mass vaccination dates back to attempts to rid 'deadly and life-threatening diseases' from the population. This was way before Big Pharma sensed an opportunity to make a killing by shaping public opinion and manipulating policy makers to promote their agenda.

So, even by the yardstick of those who believe the basic vaccine myth, immunization was supposed to be a life-saver. We have come full circle in just half a century since that myth was fed to the public. Technology has since allowed us to study microbes, the body and the way they both mesh. Now scientists can 'see' things that weren't apparent back in the 1930s and '40s. But conventional medicine has used these amazing feats to further promote the myth that germs are disease-promoting agents and that vaccines can somehow save lives.

Throughout this book, I have shown how and why vaccines have time and again caused the very diseases they are ostensibly meant to prevent. Then there are diseases and disorders produced as 'side effects' of vaccination.

Arguably the best documented among these 'side effects' is autism, a serious childhood disorder closely linked to two chemicals – thimerosal and aluminum – that were once routinely used in vaccines.

Autistic children are socially withdrawn and are unable to relate to other people. They also lack the ability to experience the normal range and depth of human emotions. Language impairment is also common, adding to their lack of communication skills. In extreme cases, autistic children exhibit repetitive actions and experience seemingly odd preoccupations.

Autism is a serious disorder and autistic individuals often need life-long supervision. Autism is sometimes considered an umbrella term for a spectrum of disorders with similar symptoms and is called Autism Spectrum Disorders (ASD).

ASD is a group of neurodevelopmental disorders, which means that behavioral development in autistic infants and children has failed to hit the usual developmental milestones because of abnormalities in the functioning of the brain and nervous system. While some scientists suggest a genetic link to autism, the causes of this disorder remain largely 'non-specific'. This means that the disease cannot be causally linked to *any* specific factors.

There is an entire body of work that has studied the pathophysiology of autism. This area focuses on abnormalities in the brain and nervous system in areas that control the functions of language, speech, emotions, expression and other 'higher functions'. It is these functions and skills that make us 'complete, whole individuals' and it is these very skills that are classically compromised by ASDs.

If genetic factors tell only half the story, circumstances in the environment comprise the other half. Of these environmental factors, vaccines play a significant role.

Many researchers, backed by hundreds of studies, believe that toxic chemicals are closely related to autism. These include pollutants in water, proximity to hazardous waste sites and even the food we eat.

A considerable amount of research has focused on chemicals such as tetrachloroethylene, trichloroethylene and trihalomethanes in drinking water, and metals such as mercury, cadmium and nickel in the atmosphere in localities where autism rates are especially high. Simple scrutiny of these chemicals reveals that the most frequently occurring chemical is mercury, a heavy metal known to cause neurological and renal or kidney damage.

As far as vaccines go, there is a huge debate on the role of a preservative called 'thimerosal' used in vaccines. Thimerosal is used as a preservative to prevent bacteria and fungi from contaminating and infecting the vaccine dose when stored for lengthy periods in vials. Thimerosal is almost 50 percent mercury, a neurotoxin that causes nerve damage to the central nervous system.

More specifically, vaccines under scrutiny for thimerosal have classically been the Hepatitis B, Hib, DTaP and MMR vaccines, all of which contain thimerosal. Research has shown that all these vaccines are closely correlated with autism and immune-related disorders.

Before we discuss thimerosal and its role in autism, there is something else we need to consider. The scientific community – and even the legal community – says it has found no 'causal link' between this mercury-laden preservative and autism. This could mean one of two things or both – a causal relationship exists but has not yet been established (studies on drugs are notoriously known to favor Big Pharma and almost always support government policies) or, at best, that a strong correlation exists.

In the latter case, the vast amount of research on thimerosal suggests that mercury, aluminum and some contaminants such as human fetal cells precipitate autism in children who are already predisposed to it. In other words, the mercury in these vaccines acts on a pre-existing neurological make-up that lends itself to autism and autism-related disorders to bring out full-blown symptoms. This means that if a child who is predisposed to autism has not been immunized with vaccines containing thimerosal, he or she would have gone through life as a normal, healthy individual who does not experience or exhibit symptoms of autism.

1. Introducing Thimerosal

Let us return to our discussion on thimerosal. Pharmaceutical manufacturers love this vaccine preservative, a synthetic chemical which, in many ways, is far more toxic than its predecessor, methylmercury hydroxide.

It is highly soluble in water, it dissolves easily on cell membranes and it has the ability to inactivate essential cell processes. Bear this in mind while reading this chapter, which dwells largely on the neurotoxic effects of this highly potent preservative.

Having said that, have you ever wondered why there has been a significant leap in the number of autism cases in the US post-1988? Could this be linked to the sudden increase in exposure to thimerosal through mandatory immunization in the Childhood Vaccination Schedule?

Until 1988, the DTaP vaccine was the only vaccine that contained thimerosal administered to infants in the US. However, in that year, the Childhood Vaccine Schedule was expanded to include other vaccines which contained this toxic preservative. Then, in 1991, it was amended and expanded once again, to include many more mercury-containing vaccines. Worse still, the modified schedule exposed even younger infants to vaccines containing thimerosal.

Which were these vaccines? In 1988, according to recommendations by the CDC, all infants born to mothers with Hepatitis B were given the Hepatitis B Immunoglobulin and the Hepatitis B vaccines within 12 hours of birth. Both these shots contained thimerosal, taking the amount of mercury injected into each infant to 37.5 micrograms (mcg).

The third mercury-laden shot was the Hib vaccine (against the hemophilus influenza Type B bacterium), which was to be administered at age 18 months. That's an additional 25 mcg of mercury, taking the total to 62.5 mcg.

Some infants were exposed to thimerosal from an additional source. These were babies born of mothers who are Rh-negative and who had been administered Rho-Gam during pregnancy. Rho-Gam is an Rh immune globulin given to these women to prevent hemolytic disease, a condition where the mother's immune system attacks fetal blood cells. This was a relatively recent development as Rho-Gam was never given to pregnant women prior to 1990.

Research shows that the brains of fetuses are more vulnerable to neurotoxins than those of adults. Neurotoxins are toxic chemicals that cause nerve damage and cell death, and mercury tops the list of chemicals that damage the brain and nervous system. Also, the younger the age, the greater the risk of neurological damage.

This type of damage destroys cells in certain areas of the brain that are linked to the classic symptoms of neurodevelopmental disorders of the type witnessed in autism spectrum disorders.

The year 1991 was a watershed – and potentially lethal – year in childhood vaccination. By then, the influence of vaccine manufacturers and their stranglehold on national health policy had increased dramatically and so had their incentives to policy makers who implemented and enforced a vaccine-heavy agenda in the US.

It is therefore no surprise that in 1991, there were some dramatic changes in the Childhood Vaccine Schedule regarding the Hepatitis B and Hib vaccines. Now infants were not only receiving more vaccines but were being given these doses at a younger age. Thus, suddenly, from a single shot to be administered within 12 hours of birth, infants were to be given two additional shots – the second when the infant was two months old and the third between six and 18 months.

The so-called rationale for the Hepatitis B 'boost' was that adults at risk of contracting Hepatitis B (intravenous drug users, regular recipients of blood transfusion and individuals practicing unsafe sex) are unlikely to get vaccinated voluntarily against the Hepatitis B virus. Therefore, vaccinating all infants was the best bet!

The Hib vaccination schedule also underwent a change. Instead of one shot at age 18 months, infants were now to be injected three more times – three shots between two and six months of age and a fourth at age 15 months. Each vial contained 25 mcg of mercury!

It was during these years – 1988 and 1991 – that autism rates as well as those of a host of other diseases such as many types of autoimmune disorders, allergic reactions and juvenile diabetes began to soar.

It was also no coincidence that scores of parents were suddenly coming forward with complaints against the DTaP and MMR (measles, mumps and rubella) vaccine as being linked to autism in their children. (We shall discuss the MMR-autism link later in this chapter)

For some parents, the following study will be useful only in hindsight but there are millions of parents who may change their minds after reading about a study conducted by researchers from the University of Pittsburgh and Thoughtful House Center for Children in Austin, Texas. These researchers administered infant rhesus macaque monkeys a series of vaccines mimicking the Childhood Vaccination Schedule recommended in the 1990s. This was a longitudinal study which used hi-tech imaging and other tests to meticulously examine and compare the brains of these test monkeys to those of monkeys that were not vaccinated. The monkeys that were vaccinated showed changes in their brains typically associated with autism while the unvaccinated monkeys' brains remained unchanged on these parameters.

What were these changes? Monkeys who had been vaccinated displayed an increase in brain volume, which has strong links to autism. They also experienced changes in the amygdala, the region of the brain closely linked to autistic disorders.

Here is something that further strengthens the link between the vaccine schedule and vaccine-makers – immunization programs invariably receive funding from vaccine manufacturers such as 'Every Child By Two', a national program set up by a voluntary agency part-funded Merck, Lederle and Connaught.

Funding public health programs and projects is a tried and tested route that Big Pharma have always taken to get an unsuspecting public to consume their products in a seemingly non-coercive way.

2. The Vaccine-Autism Link

Though there is still a lot we don't know about the human body and the immune system, a vast section of researchers is convinced that vaccines and autism are inherently linked.

By the mid-1990s, autism rates had soared so high that parents of autistic children vaccinated during the crucial 1988 to 1991 period began to publicly protest. Then, alarm bells began to ring so loudly in the early to mid-1990s that Congress passed the Food and Drug Administration Modernization Act in 1997. One of the provisions of the Act was that the FDA review the mercury content in various medical formulations.

Predictably, the FDA found that the inordinate amount of mercury being injected into infants was much higher than the permissible limit thanks to multiple doses of the Hepatitis B and Hib vaccines. These, along with the DTaP vaccine, which had long since been on the Childhood Vaccine Schedule, were exposing infants to grave health risks.

Just how much mercury was this? According to the FDA, infants were receiving 187.5 micrograms by 6 months of age or 40 percent more than they should have been receiving if you kept in mind the guidelines laid down by the Environmental Protection Agency!

The CDC, which continued to receive considerable flak over thimerosal, commissioned the Institute of Medicine to study mercury exposure through vaccines in infants and find out if there was any possible link to autism. While presenting its findings in 2004, the institute had categorically stated that it had found no 'causal link' between vaccines that contained thimerosal and autism.

Some claim the institute was coached to furnish these results. Though thimerosal had been banned from use in childhood vaccines by then, litigation over the chemical's effects continued to pile up and the CDC needed a public agency to 'dispel' these public doubts.

However, among the "adverse events" found by the institute to be "consistently linked" to the DTaP and MMR vaccines were autism and autism-spectrum disorders. There was another category which listed "secondary" autism (ever heard of a 'secondary' disease?) as an adverse event, which were autism-like symptoms caused by chronic encephalopathy (abnormalities in brain tissue) and mitochondrial disorders.

The institute also stated that it was "biologically plausible" that thimerosal could be correlated with "neurodevelopmental delays" in some children.

However, the CDC, FDA and other public health agencies focused only on the phrase "no causal link" and used it to try and calm the gullible public into believing that that there was no reason to worry about the multiple and repeated thimerosal-laden vaccines that their infants were receiving.

However, when you go behind the smokescreen, the results of this study only confirmed the correlation between thimerosal and autism. Without actually using the word 'causing' (Oh, how public agencies love to quibble over words!), the institute had only corroborated the correlation between vaccines and autistic disorders.

In addition, the CDC had also asked the institute to investigate another dimension of the vaccination debate – that vaccines caused 'neuroinflammation' and 'hyperarousal' or 'overexcitation' of the immune system.

This was suspected to have been taking place since 1988, when the number of vaccines had dramatically increased. In fact, to date, infants receive a minimum 38 doses of vaccines by the age of 18 months! (See CFS: 'New-Age Polio' in Chapter 5: Vaccine Hangover). Simply put: the VICP wondered whether infants were receiving too many vaccines.

But is not only the generalized overexcitation of the immune system that is suspected to be linked to neurological disorders. More specifically, it is certain 'contaminants' and other ingredients in vaccines which have long been associated with nerve and tissue damage.

Let me present some findings about vaccines that use live attenuated vaccines. These are vaccines that contain a live but weakened form of the virus that the vaccine allegedly offers protection from.

Scientists grow and replicate weakened forms of viruses by injecting the pathogen's basic genetic material in a host, which could be a variety of animal species. One such vaccine was the Oral Poliovirus Vaccine (OPV). Studies have found that mutations tend to aggregate or pile up with each successive vaccine and cause adverse reactions.

Also, the attenuated virus in the OPV has, on occasion, been found to recombine with the enteroviruses in the human body, returning the polio virus to its pathogenic potency. In other words, this process rekindles the weakened virus's ability to cause polio.

Another source of contamination comes from viruses present in the host that grows the attenuated virus. We have discussed SV40 contamination at length in Chapter 2: Historical Blunders. But there are many other types of genetic and viral material associated with specific vaccines. These adventitious or 'accidental' viruses come from the cell lines used to manufacture and replicate the weakened virus and from the animal sera and other biologics used in cell cultures.

For instance, Avian Leukosis Virus (ALV) and Endogenous Avian Virus (AEV) have been found in attenuated vaccines grown in chicken embryo fibroblasts. Vaccine-associated ALV and AEV are believed to have come from endogenous retroviruses in the chicken germ line.

According to a study conducted by the American Society for Microbiology and whose findings were released in 2010, researchers found human Retrovirus K or HERV-K in the MMR and Varivax vaccines. They concluded that HERV-K originated from human cell lines used to grow these viruses. This appears to support other research which suggests that certain genetic abnormalities in autistic children were linked to the presence of HERV-K in their bodies.

Some scientists have also found that the sudden rise in autism in the US correlates not only with the increase in thimerosal in childhood vaccines but also with the use of aborted fetal cells.

According to a study by the EPA, autism has increased dramatically since the 1980s, which is about the same time pharmaceutical companies began using fetal cells from aborted pregnancies on a large scale. The study correlated data from decade-long studies in the US, Denmark and Japan.

Moreover, these fetal-based cells were used in common vaccines such as the MMR vaccine. It is no coincidence that autism rates peaked in 1981, just two years after the new MMRII vaccine with fetal cells was approved and started being injected into infants on a mass scale in the US.

Autism rates also peaked in 1995, when the chickenpox vaccine was modified. This version of the vaccine now contained fetal cells. There is more. No less than 11 vaccines routinely administered in the US contain aborted fetal cells, including vaccines for polio and rabies.

3. Poisonous Preservative

As mentioned earlier, the brains of autistic children exhibit an impaired ability to process cognitive information. Autism is also associated with impaired emotional development. In addition, language and communication as well as social skills are also retarded.

This inability to effectively process, integrate and comprehend information by the brain points to either the lack of adequate development or damage to certain areas of the cerebral cortex, which controls these various functions.

This damage involves the central nervous system and is therefore neurological in nature. How does this tie in with the fact that there seems to be a statistically higher incidence of autoimmune dysfunctions – which includes enhanced autoimmunity and decreased immune function – in autistic children?

Researchers conclude that vaccines and their ingredients impact the immune system – in fact, vaccines act through the very immune system, and alter its very functioning in the process. This sometimes leads to immune dysfunction including autoimmune disorders.

Infants receiving vaccines containing mercury – including repeated doses that increase their exposure to this poisonous heavy metal at a very tender age – are thus victims of a double whammy. So if the vaccine per se is harmful enough, the mercury in some of them wreaks further damage.

This is especially true for infants, whose brains, nervous systems, immune systems and body as a whole not only works differently from that of adults but is also much more vulnerable to the dangerous effects of vaccines and their various ingredients.

But why exactly is mercury so devastating to the human body? Mercury is found in three forms – organic, inorganic and elemental. When it enters the bloodstream, this heavy metal damages the heart, brain, kidneys, lungs and immune system. The type and extent of damage depends on the type and amount of mercury that enters the bloodstream, the individual's age and the length of time for which the individual has been exposed to it.

Classically, sources of mercury poisoning have been water pollution and the fish that live in such water, mercury in teeth fillings and from the burning of coal and other products. Apart from vaccines, many over-the-counter drugs also contain thimerosal as a preservative.

Just as in autism, research has found that males are more susceptible to mercury poisoning than females, especially children. The reason infants are most vulnerable to this heavy metal is that their blood-brain barrier, which keeps harmful substances from reaching the brain, is not developed as it is in adults.

Also, as the blood-brain barrier develops, it keeps the mercury that has slipped past it from leaving, which is why it gets trapped in the brains of children. Usually, autism shows up by the age of 18 months to two years. But this slow buildup of mercury and the fact that the damaging effects of the chemical show up only later, account for the fact that many vaccinated newborn babies exhibit autistic symptoms after a delay of several months.

Another problem with mercury poisoning is that this heavy metal tends to remain in the bodies of even adults. Like all other toxins, the blood delivers it to the liver to be broken down and excreted. However, rather than detoxify the chemical, the liver routes the mercury to the bile, which then pours into the digestive tract. The mercury is then re-absorbed into the bloodstream only to circulate and cause further metabolic and neurological havoc.

Having pointed to the link between mercury, autism and autoimmunity, let us study the connection between various combinations of these three factors.

4. Autism & Autoimmunity

Research on autism and autoimmunity has found several ways in which neurological damage could lead to the appearance of autism-related symptoms. One of these ways is damage to the myelin sheath of nerves in the brain.

Every nerve cell in the body is covered with a myelin sheath, a fatty covering that helps in the conduction of the nerve impulse and that protects the nerve cell. The myelin sheath is all but absent at birth in the delicate brain of the neonate. It begins to grow gradually, starting at the fetal stage and continuing up to age 10.

It starts developing in the 'lower' areas of the brain and finally reaches the frontal lobes or 'higher' centers responsible for our ability to think, speak, communicate and feel differentiated emotions. All these functions are impaired to different degrees in autistic children.

Studies on the autism-autoimmunity link have found that many autistic children have antibodies in their blood that are believed to attack two crucial brain proteins – Myelin Basic Protein (MBP) and Neuron-Axon Filament Protein.

Please note: I personally don't agree with the interpretation that antibodies attack the cells but rather hold the opinion that the body produces these antibodies to help it heal itself and dispose of the accumulated toxins that have entered the cells and tissues as a result of vaccination. As I have already mentioned, antibodies and white blood cells are primarily involved in healing, not in fighting. This appropriate immune response obviously uses tissue inflammation to expel toxins, break down injured cells, produce scar tissue and induce as much healing as possible, given the dire situation of severe toxicity. I therefore hesitate to use the words 'autoimmune' and 'disease' in relation to autism or other so-called autoimmune diseases when it actually involves the body's wisdom of self-preservation rather than an act of self-destruction. Having said this, I will continue to use the ideas of current medical understanding to explain how vaccines are responsible for the brain damage they cause.

At the end, it doesn't really matter how we view the situation. The fact remains that dumping a cocktail of heavy metals, formaldehyde, antibiotics, antifreeze agents, foreign body parts, etc into the blood and brain of a developing child that does not stand a chance of filtering out this sludge of toxins, constitutes an assault of the highest order.

Going back to the discussion, all this means that the developing myelin sheath of the brain's nerve cells is attacked by the body itself or prevented from forming properly because of the exposure to deadly vaccine ingredients). This, in turn, damages the nerves and thus impacts the functions they control. There are many parallels between antibodies to MBP found in autistic children and in individuals with other autoimmune diseases such as systemic lupus erythematosus, thyroid disease, rheumatoid arthritis, insulin-dependent diabetes and multiple sclerosis.

And there are many reasons why this abnormality exists including genetic factors, attacks from microorganisms such as the rubella virus and cytomegalovirus infections (both these have been linked to autism), antibodies passed on from mother to fetus, and faulty immune activation.

It is the last factor that concerns us in our discussion on autism and autoimmunity – faulty immune activation caused by vaccines. Earlier in this book (See Chapter 5: *The Vaccine Hangover*), we discussed some of the ways in which vaccines set off abnormal immune responses. Moreover, the mercury present in some vaccines is one of the many ingredients associated with an autoimmune response.

The antibody-mediated immune response or antibodies against the brain may be precipitated by other ingredients and contaminants such as the adjuvant aluminum, preservatives, antibiotics (which alone contain hundreds of active ingredients such as, penicillin, bacitracin, chloramphenicol, gentamicin sulfate, neomycin sulfate, polymyxin B, oxytetracycline, kanamycin, streptomycin, sulfametrole, tosufloxacin, cycloserine, astromicin, etc) as well as foreign proteins of human and/or animal origin so abundantly present in vaccines.

Here is another way of looking at the same effect. The polio virus is believed to attack and damage the myelin sheath, which in full-blown form results in poliomyelitis. In many cases, polio causes paralysis, which in turn is the result of damage to the brain and nervous system.

Research into vaccination over the years has consistently linked vaccines to encephalitis or inflammation of the brain, which also leads to de-myelination of the nerves. The conclusion is unequivocal.

5. The Thimerosal Debate

Thimerosal has been used in various medical formulations including vaccines since the 1930s. But in the 1980s, public anxiety over vaccines and their damaging effects on children was mounting and began to spill over. This led to an increase in the number of lawsuits filed in civil courts against vaccine manufacturers, especially with regard to a possible link between the thimerosal-containing DTaP vaccine and autism.

In fact, there were more than 1,000 cases filed from 1979 to 1997, against the makers of the DtaP vaccine alone, with the largest number in a single year being 255 in 1988.

Worried that parents would stop giving their children the DtaP shot and fearing a backlash, the US government set up the National Vaccine Injury Compensation Program (VCIP) in 1988 (coinciding with the large number of vaccine-related lawsuits filed in that year).

Unofficially called the 'Vaccine Court', this legal forum was meant to be an independent legal platform for litigation regarding vaccines but the rules were very stringent. It placed the onus of proof of a 'causal link' between a vaccine and its effect on the plaintiff for the latter to receive compensation.

A decade later, the red flag went up once again, in 1997, this time from New Jersey Democrat Frank Pallone Jr., under whose jurisdiction were scores of small fishing towns, where mercury levels in fish were raising serious health concerns. Eventually, the Food and Drug Administration Modernization Act was signed into law in November 1997, which sought a review of mercury content in various foods and drugs including vaccines.

The FDA's review into the levels of mercury infants were receiving through the immunization program was made public two years later. It alerted Dr Neal Halsey, then Director of the Institute for Vaccine Safety at the Johns Hopkins School of Public Health.

Dr Halsey, who had worked with the federal vaccination program and several government health agencies, studied the data before him and went on to express his opinions publicly. He stated that he was worried that the mercury in childhood vaccines may have "caused subtle neurological impairment and learning disabilities" in the children who had received them.

Dr Halsey's statement lit a firestorm and his pro-vaccination colleagues, the FDA and other government agencies pushing the childhood vaccination program were furious. Eventually – and though no causal relationship has yet been established between thimerosal and autism – the American Academy of Pediatrics and the US Public Health Service issued a joint recommendation in 1999, stating that thimerosal be reduced or removed from all vaccines administered to infants. This was a watershed in the history of vaccination.

But there was more good news. Whether fuelled by health concerns over thimerosal or simply caving under public pressure or prompted by the desperate need to avoid further public fury, the FDA and CDC in 2001 went ahead and directed vaccine-makers to stop using thimerosal in childhood vaccines. The only ones that still contain the mercury-laden preservative are some flu shots recommended for children 6 months and older.

But even if there is a close link between thimerosal and autism, the toxic preservative is not the only neurotoxin that contributes to this serious childhood disease. Neurotoxins assault the body from many sources all at once – household cleaning agents, consumer products, processed foods and medical formulations – and it seems it's all adding up.

To illustrate just how alarming the situation is, read this: In December 2009, the CDC published a report stating that there has been a 57 percent increase in autism and autism-spectrum disorders between 2002 and 2006. That's one in every 110 children (more than 1 percent of the child population), including one in every 70 boys. At the time of writing this, one in every 94 children is diagnosed with autism. In other words, this trend continues unabated.

It is also costing the tax-payer dear. In 2007, it was estimated that $35 billion of public funds was spent on treating this disease.

6. Elaborate Cover-Up

Even as the CDC issued a joint statement asking all vaccine manufacturers to remove thimerosal from all childhood vaccines in 1999, it set in motion an almost diabolical series of events.

Never mind that they couldn't keep the dangerous preservative in vaccines; the elaborate plan was meant to whitewash the public health agencies that had been rooting for all manner of childhood vaccines. Thus, the CDC did many things to maintain the status quo as subtly but as firmly as possible.

One of the developments behind this Janus-faced act was the refusal to allow SmithKline Beecham to manufacture a DTaP vaccine that was free of thimerosal. After the CDC directive to pharmaceutical companies, the vaccine maker had told the government health agency in July 1999 that it was prepared to manufacture DTaP vaccines that did not contain thimerosal. The company said it could start manufacturing these modified vaccines immediately and produce enough stocks to last till mid-2000, by which time other vaccine-makers would be ready with further stocks.

At the time, infants were receiving three DTaP shots – at 2, 4 and 6 months of age – each containing 25 mcg of thimerosal.

Shockingly, five months later, the CDC turned down this offer! Government officials privately conceded that there were many reasons for this inexplicable decision. One, the CDC did not want to jeopardize its vaccine program. Two, in the face of the flak it was receiving, it wanted to save face. Three, it didn't want to upset its 'friends and associates' in the vaccine industry nor subject vaccine manufacturers to exorbitant costs that making and mass marketing a modified vaccine would entail.

But the fourth reason seems to be the most compelling. It appears that the World Health Organization feared that banning thimerosal in the US would jeopardize their mass immunization programs in developing countries. Eventually, the CDC had to throw in the towel. In a statement in July 2000, it was forced to state that no childhood vaccines would contain thimerosal by early 2001.

However, a month before it issued this statement, the CDC orchestrated a secret cover-up on thimerosal that shook the medical fraternity three years later when details leaked. The venue: Simpsonwood in Norcross, Georgia. The date: June 2000. The convenor: the CDC. The players: senior government officials, scientists from the CDC and FDA, vaccine specialists from the WHO, specialists in the fields of autism, pediatrics, toxicology, epidemiology and vaccines, and representatives of every major vaccine maker, including GlaxoSmithKline, Merck, Wyeth and Aventis Pasteur.

There were no public announcements and the conference had been kept under wraps from the media. Participation at this secluded location was by invitation only. Fifty-two participants turned up, participants who were told that the discussions and documents at the meetings were 'classified'.

Called the 'Scientific Review of Vaccine Safety Datalink Information', the conclave had a single-point agenda: to discuss the scare thimerosal had sparked in the public and medical community – and ways to douse the fire stoked by a study on the devastating effects of vaccine preservative and its possible link to autism. Ironically, the study had been conducted by Dr Thomas Verstraeten, a CDC epidemiologist!

The study had been ordered in 1997, when Congress passed a resolution asking the FDA to review the use of thimerosal in all biologics including vaccines. Verstraeten had analyzed the CDC's database which included the medical records of 100,000 children and discussed his findings at the Simpsonwood conference. His study had suggested that there was a strong link between thimerosal and neurological disorders in children.

What followed for the next two days were discussions on how to keep Verstraeten's findings from the public. Thanks to the Freedom of Information Act, details of the meetings eventually entered public domain, leaving Americans shocked that their watchdogs of public health and safety had sought to hush things up rather than take steps to undo the damage that had already been done to millions of children.

Verstraeten himself had said he was "stunned" at what the data presented. Other scientists were worried that the data at the CDC's disposal would provide fodder for countless lawsuits should it fall into public domain.

After the secret conclave, the CDC set in motion a series of measures for immediate damage-control. One, it withheld Verstraeten's findings, publicly claiming that the original data was lost. Two, the agency commissioned another study, by the Institute of Medicine (discussed earlier in this chapter), to counter what Verstraeten had found. Three, the CDC handed over its vast database to a private agency, thus taking its damning thimerosal-related data out of the purview of the Freedom of Information Act.

And four, Verstraeten was forced to 'rework' his findings and publish these revised results in 2003. These findings, predictably, claimed there was no link whatsoever between the mercury-containing preservative and autism. But here's another twist: By the time Verstraeten published his revised results, the former senior CDC epidemiologist had thrown in his lot with Big Pharma and was working with GlaxoSmithKline!

Apart from wanting to 'save face', the CDC and FDA had been keen to protect the interests – mainly financial – of vaccine-makers. Hence, when the FDA and CDC were forced to direct pharmaceutical companies to stop using thimerosal in their vaccines, they bought up stocks of the 'damaging' vaccines and through the WHO dumped them in developing countries for their immunization programs. What remained with vaccine-makers continued to be administered to American children till stocks finally ran out.

7. Merck's Dirty Secret

Almost an entire decade before vaccine-makers had to stop using thimerosal in children's vaccines, Merck was aware that its vaccines were exposing infants to mercury that was 87 times more than permissible levels.

This shocking truth is contained in a confidential memo written in 1991 by Dr Maurice Hilleman, one of the creators of Merck's vaccine programs and a retired senior vice-president of the company. The memo was addressed to the then chief of the company's vaccine division, Dr Gordon Douglas.

Dr Hilleman had raised concerns about the company's vaccines because Sweden and some other Scandanavian countries had just banned the use of thimerosal in vaccines. Hence, to be able to compete in the Scandanavian market, Merck would have to manufacture vaccines that were free of thimerosal, Dr Hilleman had pointed out.

In the memo, running into seven pages, the senior vaccinologist had presented an analysis of mercury exposure in American infants through vaccines. He said "it would be reasonable to conclude that it (thimerosal) should be eliminated from use in vaccines for children".

Ironically, the leaked Hilleman memo was written at same time that the Childhood Vaccine Schedule had just included several new vaccines for infants, including some with generous doses of thimerosal.

Needless to say, the memo was ignored by Merck, who turned a blind eye mounting evidence of the correlation between mercury and neurological disorders and sought refuge behind the fact that no undisputable 'causal link' could be established.

When a Texan family who was suing Merck confronted the company with a copy of Hilleman's memo, the pharma major merely shrugged it off. They claimed that the copying service responsible for photocopying evidence for the case had 'forgotten' to copy the controversial memo along with some other documents!

The solution would have been easy – all that Merck and other vaccine-makers needed to do was switch to making single-dose vaccines as only multi-dose vaccines, which were being routinely administered to infants, required to contain the preservative.

But there was a hitch – this would have seriously impacted bottom lines as it costs significantly more to manufacture smaller, single-dose vaccines. This, in turn, would have negatively impacted vaccine sales to developing countries, where pharma majors such as Merck were regularly dumping their controversial vials.

So pharma majors in the US continued to make multi-dose vaccines even as the federal authorities kept introducing more and more shots into the Childhood Vaccine Schedule. Till the axe fell in 1999 and thimerosal was banned from being used in pediatric vaccines.

But Merck is not the only pharmaceutical company accused of hiding shocking secrets. Eli Lilly, who introduced thimerosal to the world of pharmaceuticals in the 1920s and began selling it commercially on a large scale in the 1940s, harbors an equally dark secret.

Confidential communication reveals that the international pharma major was aware that its preservative could cause serious damage. More than 20 patients tested with thimerosal back in the 1930s died soon after they were tested with the chemical. Yet Eli Lilly claimed the chemical was safe for human beings when it published the results of its clinical trials. Five years later, when a rival pharmaceutical company pointed out that Eli Lilly's studies did not gel with theirs, Eli Lilly ignored the cautionary statement.

Despite international concerns over thimerosal, the preservative is still used in many over-the-counter drugs and cosmetics in the US. According to some researchers, countries that receive vaccines from the US have experienced a corresponding surge in autism rates, including China. Where the disease was once non-existent in the Asian country before 1999, when US vaccines made their way into the country, China is now estimated to have close to 2 million autistic children.

Other countries receiving vaccines made in the US have been similarly affected. These include countries in South America, Asia and Africa.

But let's not kid ourselves. Big Pharma is not concerned about human health. They have systematically and effectively worked on the human psyche to push the myth that vaccines are a mandatory rite of passage. Perhaps the bigger irony is that US public health agencies and the WHO still take refuge behind hackneyed line that's fast wearing thin, that "the vaccine-autism issue is still open to debate".

8. Landmark Litigation

After a public furor created by the suspicion that the DTaP vaccine caused Sudden Infant Death Syndrome and other adverse events, the US Department of Health established the Vaccine Court in 1988. The court was meant to adjudicate cases where families of individuals alleged that vaccines had caused injury, illness or death to their children.

Though the burden of proof of a causal link between the vaccine and the plaintiff's symptoms rested squarely on the plaintiff, hundreds of cases have been decided in their favor.

But perhaps no vaccine has attracted as much legal attention as the MMR vaccine, which contains mercury-laden thimerosal. There are, in fact, around 5,000 autism-related lawsuits pending adjudication and appeal in various US courts since 2002.

However, the year 2007 was a watershed in the history of thimerosal-related litigation. It was then that the Vaccine Court began hearings in nine test cases based on three hypotheses in the famous Omnibus Autism Proceedings.

Cases were selected and categorized on the basis of three assumptions: that a combination of the MMR vaccine and thimerosal cause autism; that thimerosal alone causes autism; and that the MMR vaccine alone causes autism. Since then, many cases have been heard, dismissed and decided in favor of the plaintiffs. One of these, the Hannah Poling case of 2008, was especially pathbreaking.

Hannah Poling had received five vaccines for nine diseases in a single day when she was 19 months old in 2000. These were vaccines for measles, mumps, rubella, varicella, diphtheria, pertussis, tetanus, polio and Haemophilus influenzae.

Just days later, the normal, healthy, bubbly child grew lethargic, irritable and feverish and stopped speaking. She also began to experience seizures and exhibit repetitive behavior typical of autism.

In other words, almost overnight, Hannah began to show symptoms of an autism spectrum disorder. Some experts call this 'regressive autism' as her symptoms showed up and regress after the child began to achieve her normal developmental milestones.

Hannah was diagnosed as suffering from 'encephalopathy', the generalized medical term for 'brain disease'. She was also found to be suffering from a mitochondrial disorder, something not often found in autistic children.

Then, abruptly in 2008, the case was taken off the Vaccine Court's test-case schedule when the federal government conceded the lawsuit and decided to award the family compensation. This was a landmark decision for parents of children who had filed autism-related lawsuits as the Polings were not asked to prove a causal link between autism and the thimerosal-laden vaccines the child had received.

The Department of Justice decreed that the Polings should receive compensation because "the vaccinations had significantly aggravated an underlying mitochondrial disorder and manifested as a regressive encephalopathy with features of autism spectrum disorder."

Not only had the ruling been given in spite of the absence of the much-argued and much-hyped 'causal link', it also confirmed something a section of researchers had been arguing for years – that vaccines and the thimerosal in many of them can precipitate serious disorders such as autism in children predisposed to them but who would not have developed symptoms had they not been vaccinated.

Another significant case decided by the Vaccine Court in favor of the plaintiff is that of 10-year-old old Bailey Banks. The case was decided in June 2007, when the court ruled that the family had indeed shown that the MMR vaccine young Bailey had received was responsible for his disorder.

Bailey had been diagnosed with Pervasive Developmental Disorder or PDD, which is one of many Autism Spectrum Disorders.

The court concluded that the plaintiff had demonstrated that the MMR vaccine had led to a brain inflammation illness called Acute Disseminated Encephalomyelitis or ADEM and this had led to PDD.

The court has decided many more cases in favor of distressed families whose children began to show symptoms of ASD after being immunized according to the government's schedule. In fact, investigative reporting has revealed that since the court was set up in 1988, it has awarded millions of dollars to more than 1,300 families in cases of brain damage from vaccines alone.

9. To Vaccinate Or Not To Vaccinate?

No discussion on autism and vaccines can be complete without mentioning Dr Andrew Wakefield, whose research into a link between the MMR vaccine and the disorder first ignited fears over a possible link between the two.

Dr Wakefield was with London's Royal Free Hospital back then and in 1998 he published a paper in the Lancet stating that the MMR vaccine triggered autism. Dr Wakefield, a British doctor now living in the US, was investigated by the British medical establishment for 12 long years.

His work has since been discredited as being unethical, his methods trashed and his medical license revoked. But if he hadn't raised suspicions then, the MMR vaccine's potential to precipitate autism-related disorders may not have received the attention it deserved.

Dr Wakefield had also alleged that the MMR vaccine has never undergone proper safety tests and that initial safety checks lasted only four weeks. After the publication of Dr Wakefield's paper in 1998, vaccination rates for MMR in the UK plummeted and the measles rate soared. The doctor's paper also prompted a series of medical studies whose findings have been published in various medical journals, refuting, denying and supporting an autism-MMR link, in the decade that followed.

However, the medical fraternity is still where it all began – no 'causal link' but overwhelming evidence of a correlation between this spectrum of disorders linked to mercury-containing vaccines.

As the debate over vaccines and their damaging effects continues, the fact is that parents in the US are increasingly questioning whether vaccines – at least so many of them – are necessary at all.

According to the study, based on records and interviews of parents of almost 9,000 children aged below 3 years and conducted through the CDC's National Immunization Survey, 39 percent of parents had delayed or refused to immunize their children. This compared with 22 percent in 2003.

Parents surveyed felt the government schedule mandated simply too many doses of vaccines. Vaccine side effects including autism were cited as another reason for their skepticism. Some even wondered whether vaccines were effective at all.

On a different note, the National Institutes of Mental Health has concluded that it is essential that pregnant women have enough Vitamin D to ensure proper development of their fetus's brains. It is equally important for the proper development of a child brain's to have enough Vitamin D after it is born. Since the child doesn't get Vitamin D from breast milk, the only natural way to obtain it is through sunlight, just as nature intended it.

Even moderate sun exposure helps ensure proper brain development. Unfortunately, sun-avoidance has increased dramatically in the last 20 years, ever since the medical community started warning about the dangers of sun exposure. Far fewer parents now expose their babies to the sun, and if they do, the babies are often given sunscreens and even sunglasses to wear! Pediatricians go as far as to warn parents to keep their infants out of the sun for at least the first six months.

The Vitamin D receptors appear in a wide variety of brain tissue early in the development of a baby and, activated Vitamin D receptors increase nerve growth in the brain. If you have an autistic child, make sure he/she spends several hours a day outdoors, and if it is warm, without clothes, so all the skin can receive this valuable treatment.

Vitamin D manages to balance the immune response and ensures that the immune system does not overreact and end up causing an unstoppable cycle of inflammation. It also prevents infection and makes vaccination unnecessary. Vitamin D serves as the ultimate natural vaccine against all infectious diseases, and no genetic mutation of germs can ever outsmart the protective mechanisms set into place by this powerful steroid hormone.

You will never learn the truth about the astonishing benefits of vitamin D from the pharmaceutical companies, the FDA, the CDC, and others who have a vested interest in keeping the sickness industry going. The dire warnings about potentially lethal effects caused by the sun were issued by leaders of the medical industry at about the same time when the then dying vaccine industry needed a 'booster vaccine'. By telling the masses that the sun was dangerous, more and more people became vitamin D deficient and found themselves in need of (costly) medical treatment for dozens of common diseases.

Now that almost the entire population is vitamin D deficient, including infants, the sickness industry and vaccine-makers are thriving like never before. Autism, Alzheimer's disease and cancer are among the best revenue-generating diseases. It would be naïve to believe that the medical industry and its guardians, the FDA, CDC and WHO would encourage or allow medical science to find a cure for these diseases.

Scientific studies show that vitamin D can prevent 70 percent of all cancers, but you will not hear these health protective agencies recommend that you spend significant lengths of time out in the sun without sun protection in order to replenish your vitamin D stores in the body. According to the FDA and contrary to the hundreds of scientific peer-reviewed studies done on vitamin D, this hormone which is known to regulate over 2,000 genes "has no beneficial biological effects in the human body." (Read my book, Heal Yourself with Sunlight, to learn how this essential element of nature positively influences our health and wellbeing, perhaps more than any other)

Chapter 7

Swine Flu - The Pandemic That Didn't Pan Out!

December 22, 2009 was a red-letter day for vaccine manufacturers. They couldn't have asked for more. Splashed across newspaper pages, websites and television channels was an image of US President Barrack Obama rolling up his sleeve to receive his swine flu shot. It took just a couple of seconds to get the jab but in that instant, the US President became a poster boy for vaccine-makers. With that sort of endorsement, could the likes of vaccine majors GlaxoSmithKline, Novartis, Sanofi Pasteur, Baxter, CSL and Medimmune have asked for more?

Ever since swine flu made its appearance in Mexico and shortly thereafter in the US, there have been lurking suspicions that the virus was fabricated in the laboratory. Conspiracy theories have flourished since mid-2009 but there is one aspect to this thriller-type plot that no one can deny – the shocking Baxter 'mix-up'.

This colossal 'mistake' came to light when experimental ferrets contracted a deadly avian flu in labs in the Czech Republic in early 2009. Further probing revealed that the vaccine administered to the ferrets was the H3N2 seasonal flu vaccine meant to be sold in the market in the winter of 2009. It had been shipped to the Czech lab by the US-based Baxter International's Austrian arm. It turned out that identical shipments had been sent to labs in Germany, Slovenia and 16 other countries as well.

If that wasn't scary enough, the crux of the plot was that Baxter's flu vaccines were contaminated or mixed with strains of the deadly H5N1 avian flu virus, which has a death rate of 60 percent. Was the 'contamination' accidental? If not, were the wrong shipments accidentally sent to these labs?

Baxter couldn't wriggle out of this one. If the contamination was not accidental, the question is: was the vaccine maker preparing a biological weapon of mass destruction? If the shipments were intended for their respective destinations, what where the recipients meant to do with the lethal biological material? If indeed it was a mistake, how did Baxter go unpunished? And how did such deadly genetic material slip past the multiple checks that have been in place at transit points post-9/11?

Some critics have wondered whether Baxter was part of a global conspiracy to deliberately spark a bird flu pandemic in the human population. Remember how the avian flu or bird flu turned out to be a damp squib in 2003?

Was there a plot at work to make sure a pandemic hit home (causing millions of human fatalities) this time? Was Baxter part of a global depopulation conspiracy, something that has been at the centre of the World Health Organization's (WHO) 'humanitarian work' for decades?

One of the suspicions is that Baxter, who had already manufactured a vaccine against H5N1, was deliberately trying to spark a pandemic to hike sales of its vaccine against the deadly bird flu. If this seems like a simplistic assumption, remember, no drug maker acts on its own. They are always part of a much larger plan where profits go to various quarters including politicians, key office-bearers of public health agencies and global health organizations.

1. Vaccines As Vehicles

What better way to spread a pandemic than to piggy-back it on a virus responsible for one of the most contagious diseases on earth – influenza? If Baxter had succeeded in unleashing the lethal H5N1 virus along with the seasonal flu virus, the world would have become a veritable laboratory.

Millions of people would have become incubators for a process called 'reassortment', a process whereby genetic material of two (or more) strains of a virus mix to eventually produce a new strain. Out there among billions of people and spreading rapidly, the process of reassortment would have almost definitely led to a mutant influenza virus strain that contained elements of the deadly avian flu.

But this is no surprise. Vaccines have been used as a vehicle to spread deadly diseases ever since they were invented. The first major scandal broke when it was discovered that the Inactivated Polio Vaccine had been contaminated with the SV40 virus (See Chapter 2: Historical Blunders) and had been used in mass immunization programs between 1955 and 1963. The vaccine is suspected to have since caused cancers in the bones, brain and other organs in human beings and its effects are still being felt by individuals immunized during those times.

Next, the Hepatitis B vaccine was used as a vehicle to introduce the HIV virus into unsuspecting homosexual males in Manhattan in the 1980s. (See Chapter 3: Is There A Conspiracy?) By the time this was discovered, it was too late.

At the same time that the HIV virus was introduced to millions of people through the Hepatitis B vaccine, another company was brewing a genetic time bomb with full knowledge of its consequences. The company was Bayer, who along with two other companies including Baxter (why aren't we surprised?), had used blood plasma from high-risk donors including homosexual males and prison inmates to make a concentrate that would treat hemophiliacs.

Bayer's Factor VIII was an injectable drug administered to hemophiliacs to aid blood clotting. In its haste to obtain the blood plasma required to prepare its formulation, Bayer had broken federal laws requiring the company to screen out donors with viral hepatitis. Blood plasma was thus drawn from around 10,000 high-risk donors who were paid for their services in the late 1980s.

Since the HIV virus had already been circulating among high-risk groups, who had been deliberately targeted for the HIV virus, Bayer's plasma too contained the deadly HIV virus. As a result, the virus was transmitted to around 10,000 hemophiliacs in the US through Bayer's Factor VIII which had been thus contaminated.

While the scandal was chilling enough, further investigations revealed that Bayer had been aware of its contaminated product but chose to keep quiet. When Factor VIII was pulled off the market and the company developed a newer version of the drug (heat-treated to kill the HIV virus in it), Bayer sold the older version of the product to countries in Europe, Asia and Latin America, where thousands of hemophiliac children contracted the HIV virus through the 'life-saving' drug.

Bayer had the audacity to write to distributors in these countries, saying that AIDS was "the center of irrational response in many countries" and they need not be wary of its drug!

Also, classified internal documents sourced from the company reveal that Bayer had colluded with the FDA to cover up the scandal. Though not one Bayer executive has faced charges, a French health official did go to jail for allowing the sale and distribution of Bayer's tainted drug.

But pharma companies and public health agencies are not known to have a conscience. Hence it was no surprise when it emerged in

April 2009 that Baxter was among the elite caucus of vaccine manufacturers contracted to make the much sought-after swine flu vaccine. And if public memory is short, it seems the US federal authorities were suffering from an acute case of amnesia – the announcement came less than two months after the Baxter avian flu conspiracy.

And this wasn't the first time the American vaccine company had been involved in efforts to help prevent (or create?) epidemics, pandemics and thwart threats of bioterrorism.

Here is Baxter's illustrious track record in this department:

- Smallpox: After the September 11, 2001 tragedy, the company supplied stockpiles of a smallpox vaccine. It did this in collaboration with UK-based biotech company Acambis.

- SARS: After the outbreak of Severe Acute Respiratory Syndrome (SARS) in 2003, the US government contracted Baxter to produce a vaccine against this disease.

- Nerve Poisons: In 2005, Baxter was one of two firms who worked on a "plasma-based therapeutic agent targeted for use in individuals who may be exposed to nerve gas poisons".

- Flu Vaccines: In 2006 (three years before the swine flu outbreak), the British government said it had planned to vaccinate every single individual in the country with vaccines made by Baxter in case of a flu pandemic.

The vaccine maker's next windfall came from the swine flu 'pandemic'. Baxter definitely has friends in high government offices in major developed countries. How else did it land these prestigious research and commercial projects?

And these are only its high-profile mandates that have been made public. Baxter has also been the beneficiary of massive government funding. For instance, in 2006, the Bush administration had gifted $1 billion to vaccine manufacturers including Baxter to hasten production of their vaccines. Baxter in particular was awarded a five-year contract to develop both seasonal and pandemic vaccines.

2. WHO Is To Blame?

The avian flu epidemic that never was wasn't the only elaborate and carefully orchestrated vaccination plan that went horribly wrong. The 2009 swine flu 'pandemic' is another example.

Of the millions of deaths predicted, there were only 14,000-odd fatalities the world over in the wake of the 2009 swine flu outbreak. Of these, 12,000 were initially assumed to have been in the US, but it turned out to be just a fraction of that.

So just how far off the mark was the virus?

The WHO's website states that seasonal flu is responsible for 250,000 to 500,000 deaths a year worldwide (36,000 in the US). With the H1N1 virus claiming 14,000-odd lives globally, the worldwide swine flu toll is less than half the number of people who die of seasonal flu in the US every year. For vaccine-makers and their political patrons, how very embarrassing!

So when the WHO and US public health agencies (always working in tandem with each other) realized that the 'pandemic' had turned out to be a damp squib, they had to do something, and do it quick! The easiest solution to save face and confuse the public was to resort to juggling with semantics. So the WHO, high priest of every aspect of global health/disease, simply changed its definition of a 'pandemic'!

This is how the WHO earlier defined an 'influenza pandemic' on its official website. *"An influenza pandemic occurs when a new influenza virus appears against which the human population has no immunity, resulting in several simultaneous epidemics worldwide* **with enormous numbers of deaths and illness.** *With the increase in global transport and communications, as well as urbanization and overcrowded conditions, epidemics due the new influenza virus are likely to quickly take hold around the world."*

Now here's the reworded 'influenza pandemic' definition. *"A disease epidemic occurs when there are more cases of that disease than normal. A pandemic is a worldwide epidemic of a disease. An influenza pandemic may occur when a new influenza virus appears against which the human population has no immunity. With the increase in global transport, as well as urbanization and overcrowded conditions in some areas, epidemics due to a new influenza virus are likely to take hold around the world, and become a pandemic faster than before. WHO has defined the phases of a pandemic to provide a global framework to aid countries in pandemic preparedness and response planning.* **Pandemics can be either mild or severe in the** *illness and deaths they cause, and the severity of a pandemic can change over the course of that pandemic."*

Note the two critical changes. One, the second definition makes no mention of 'enormous numbers of deaths' and two, it slipped in the phrase 'pandemics can be either mild or severe'.

It is no coincidence that the definition changed *after* the WHO took note of the pattern in the outbreak. And, to explain why the so-called pandemic wasn't (thankfully) as disastrous as the agency had hoped, it conveniently added in its new definition that "the severity can change over the course of that pandemic"!

The only single factor the WHO based its definition of a pandemic on was the transmissibility of the virus (no more or less than the seasonal flu virus), not its severity or potential to be lethal.

3. Billions Down The Drain

In the aftermath of the scare and the millions of people who got themselves vaccinated or were forced to by bully governments, here is some serious number-crunching.

Data available as of April 2010 suggests that just six months after the mad scramble to get pharma to save millions of people from swine flu, just over half these 'life-saving' vaccines were actually administered and large quantities of them were in danger of expiring i.e. of the 229 million doses of H1N1 vaccines purchased by the US government, only 91 million doses were administered to an unsuspecting population by February 2010. A whopping 71 million doses were slated to be destroyed as they exceeded their expiry date; and millions of unused doses were shipped to developing countries.

Needless to say, to make good use of most of the unused vaccines, the US health agencies have decided to combine them with the new regular flu vaccines and offer Americans "double" protection of season or the 2010 flu, just in case the swine flu makes a comeback.

This whole fiasco has, of course, come at a huge cost to the tax-payer as the US government paid four vaccine-makers $1.6 billion to make H1N1 vaccines in 2009. In France alone, the government had purchased 94 million doses of vaccines at a cost of $734 million but less than 10 percent of the population chose to get vaccinated.

Of course, governments and agencies like the WHO don't make colossal mathematical 'mistakes'. When numbers like these don't add up, there's usually a perfectly logical explanation and sometimes, someone succeeds in belling the cat.

172

In January 2010, German politician and chairman of the Council of Europe's Health Committee, Wolfgang Wodarg, minced no words when he publicly alleged that global health agencies had intentionally whipped up fears of a global pandemic at the behest of vaccine manufacturers, the sole motive being economic gain. The Council of Europe, a not-for-profit organization and human rights watchdog body, then proceeded to take the WHO to task in a report it published in June 2010.

Wodarg, a doctor himself, accused Big Pharma of coaxing public health agencies to press the panic button to declare a false pandemic. Tracing the conspiracy back to Mexico, to the epicenter of the swine flu epidemic in 2009, he alleged that a hundred-odd flu cases had been declared as a 'new pandemic' even though there was no scientific evidence for doing so.

Faced with such scathing criticism, the WHO went into damage-control mode and announced in April 2010 that it would initiate an investigation into the matter. This inquiry would ostensibly investigate whether the pandemic had been mishandled in the agency's failure to inform the public about the uncertainties of the pandemic.

The WHO's top influenza expert Keiji Fukuda was forced to admit that the H1N1 virus was not as deadly as initially perceived. But he blamed the confusion on two factors: One, the confusing parameters used to declare a pandemic and two, the H5N1 bird flu virus! Believe it or not but in a public statement, Fukuda said that the H5N1 bird flu virus had killed more than half the number of people it had infected since 2003 and this had "injected a high level of fear about the next pandemic".

He also said that faced with the sudden nature of the 2009 outbreak and the newness of the H1N1 strain that had led to the 'pandemic', public health agencies and experts were initially not sure whether a single dose of the vaccine would work. The vaccination program had been designed around two doses per head, which accounted for the large number of doses that had been ordered (much to the glee of vaccine-makers).

Even as the WHO announced its lofty claim to investigate the severity of the epidemic (we all know how these inquiries are engineered to whitewash reputations), millions of doses of unused swine flu vaccines were being magnanimously dispatched to developing countries. There are 95 nations listed as beneficiaries.

But we all know that magnanimity is not among the US government's virtues. (See Chapter 3: Is There A Conspiracy?)

But what happens when the numbers don't add up? It seems once the damage was done by the hype stirred up by the WHO, individual governments, public health agencies and a willing media, these perpetrators needed to cover their tracks. And that meant a halt to generating damaging data.

That is why the CDC did an inexplicable turnaround in July 2009 only four months after the 'deadly pandemic' had broken and only a month after it was raised to a 'Level 6 pandemic'.

In a communication to individual states dated July 24, 2009, the CDC had instructed each state and all public health agencies to stop counting H1N1 cases and stop turning in data on the swine flu! Note, this was at the height of the pandemic panic.

Here's the text of the notice: "Attached are the Q&As that will be posted on the CDC website tomorrow explaining why CDC is no longer reporting case counts for novel H1N1. CDC would have liked to have run these by you for input but unfortunately there was not enough time before these needed to be posted."

The CDC led the states to believe that there was no point counting swine flu cases when it had already been proved that there was an epidemic out there sweeping the world. But the truth is that most of the flu cases out there had not tested positive for swine flu or even flu at all!

How's that? Well, most of those who thought they had the flu indeed exhibited flu-like symptoms but, at best, these flu-like symptoms were probably caused by an upper respiratory tract illness or other similar infections. The culprit was therefore not the much-maligned H1N1 virus but some other pathogen!

The fact is that many pathogens turn virulent in cycles relating to the seasons and many of these provoke symptoms that resemble the flu. According to experts, there are as many as 150 and 200 infectious pathogens such as parainfluenza, adenovirus and rhinovirus, coronavirus and pneumonia that produce flu-like symptoms. Others include less common microbes such as bocavirus which causes bronchitis and pneumonia in children and metapneumovirus, which is responsible for around 5 percent of all flu-related illnesses.

So how do we know that most of those dreaded swine flu cases were not swine flu at all? The massive CDC cover-up was unearthed by Sharyl Attkisson, investigative news reporter for the US television channel CBS. The facts she had used to arrive at her conclusions had come from statistics obtained under the Freedom of Information Act, and the statistics had come from individual states which had tested samples turned in by physicians who, in turn, had surrendered samples from suspected swine flu cases that walked into their clinics. These are Attkisson's shocking findings:

- In Florida, 83 percent of specimens suspected to be swine flu were negative for all types of flu when tested.
- In California, 86 percent of suspected H1N1 specimens were not swine flu or any flu. Only 2 percent were confirmed swine flu.
- In Alaska, 93 percent of suspected swine flu specimens were negative for all types of flu. Only 1 percent was H1N1 flu.

These were devastating conclusions for the CDC, FDA and US government, which had gone all out to fabricate and market the swine flu 'pandemic'. Here's but one example of how the outbreak was enthusiastically blown out of proportion.

After all the hype and hoopla, it transpired that the swine flu toll as reported by the media was often based on incidents like this one at Georgetown University in Washington DC. Media reports in September 2009 stated that the swine flu virus had infected 250 students at this university. If this were indeed true, it would have been deadly serious. It turned out that the figure was based on the number of panicky students who had approached the students' health center and/or called the doctor-on-call to report flu-like symptoms!

4. Money Makes The Virus Go Round!

We discussed the allegations made by Wolfgang Wodarg earlier in this chapter. What you are about to read confirms the German doctor's allegations. It is an article published in a scientific journal that has nailed the WHO, no less.

Published in the *BMJ (British Medical Journal)* on June 4, 2010, the article states that three of the 22 scientists on the panel that had drawn up the WHO influenza pandemic guidelines in 2004 were on the payroll of key vaccine-makers.

Worse still (and why doesn't this surprise us?), the world body had not disclosed this conflict of interest and went on to accept their recommendations which have subsequently led these very companies to reap billions of dollars thanks to these very guidelines, which advised governments to buy (stockpile) antiviral drugs to counter flu pandemics that may arise.

In some stellar investigative work by the authors of the *BMJ*, (which included the London-based Bureau of Investigative Journalism, a non-profit-organization), the following evidence was provided against the three key players:

Prof Fred Hayden: His consultancy and lectures were being sponsored by Swiss vaccine maker Hoffman-La Roche (maker of Tamiflu) and GlaxoSmithKline (Relenza) at the time he wrote his now-famous guidelines on antiviral drugs for the WHO.

It gets even murkier. Turns out Prof Hayden was also one of the lead researchers of a study funded by Roche. Not surprisingly, his guidelines claimed that Tamiflu would cut hospitalizations from the flu virus by as much as 60 percent. The company went on to reap millions from the sale of its drug. But then that is history now.

Dr Arnold Monto: He wrote the WHO annex on the use of vaccines during pandemics. During this time, Dr Monto had accepted money from both Roche and GlaxoSmithKline for his own consultancy work.

Prof Karl Nicholson: He was an integral advisor to the WHO on pandemic influenza. Like Hayden and Monto, he too had been funded by both Roche and GlaxoSmithKline in the past.

Four days after the *BMJ* published its damning article, the WHO issued a weak rejoinder which stated that when it had recruited the experts onto the panel, it had weighed their privacy against "the robustness of guidelines" which had been subjected to external review.

According to WHO Director-General Margaret Chan, the agency's decisions had "not for a second" been influenced by commercial interests or any ties the scientists had to the pharmaceutical industry. Like most official denials, this one too couldn't actually prove otherwise.

Now allow me to illustrate exactly how a 'recommendation' directly translates into profits for a pharma company. The WHO's 2004 guidelines on pandemic flu clearly advise: **"Countries that are considering the use of antivirals as part of their pandemic response will need to stockpile in advance."**

Vaccine-makers and governments who have a cozy symbiotic relationship with vaccine manufacturers couldn't get a more blatant mandate than this. Pretending to be seized with apprehension and purporting to be adequately forearmed, public health agencies in various countries across the world immediately began buying Tamiflu and other antiviral drugs in bulk – five whole years before the swine flu 'pandemic' broke.

How else do you explain that some of the world's biggest vaccine-makers had filed for swine flu vaccine patents even *before* the outbreak in April 2009? Vaccine researchers have dug out the following facts:

Baxter had filed Vaccine Patent Application US 2009/0060950 A1 as early as August 2008 and had published this in March of 2009. Then, Novartis had filed its own patent, US 20090047353 A1, on November 4, 2005. The patent was granted by the US Patent Office on February 19, 2009.

Interestingly, four years before the 2009 'pandemic', Novartis had devised a 'Split Influenza Vaccine', which effectively combines multiple virus strains. (The 2009 swine flu virus is said to contain four viral strains, a split-influenza vaccine!)

According to some experts, after the WHO guidelines were announced, pharmaceutical companies reeled in more than $7 billion as governments stockpiled vaccines. The UK, for instance, which apprehended 65,000 deaths from a flu pandemic (there were eventually 400 fatalities), placed an initial order for 14.6 million doses of Tamiflu in 2005. The government has since ordered an investigation into the $232 million spent by its public health agency, the National Health Service, to determine just how much this panic buying cost the taxpayer.

While on the subject of transparency, the *BMJ* has pointed to another 'secret' group which it alleges has been steering the 2009 swine flu 'pandemic'. This is a 16-member group set up by the WHO to guide it on all aspects of the so-called pandemic, including what emergency levels to declare and when to declare that the 'pandemic' was over.

The international body has not disclosed the identities of these 16 members, ostensibly to protect them from the reach of industry. The truth is that the members are on that panel *because* of their links with industry and it would be no surprise if there were representatives of the major vaccine-makers involved in the swine-flu 'pandemic' in that group as well.

5. They Had A Premonition

So how come all the hype and panic about swine flu years before the virus surfaced full-blown? How did the WHO know half a decade in advance that there would be an influenza 'pandemic' if it wasn't engineered?

The origins of the panic date back to the bird flu or avian flu outbreak of 2003. This pandemic – mainly among birds, not human beings – broke out in many Asian countries, where millions of infected poultry died from the H5N1 strain of the Type A influenza family of viruses. Millions more had to be culled so that they would not be consumed by the human population. And herein lies the rub: there were only 40 suspected human deaths from bird flu that year. The virus simply refused to cooperate!

What were vaccine-makers and governments across developing countries supposed to do with the antiviral drugs they had stockpiled during the bird flu epidemic? For those in high places, the answer was obvious: scare up a pandemic.

Hence, a year after countries like Vietnam, South Korea and Thailand culled their poultry, the WHO announced its guidelines for an influenza pandemic. Conveniently, the WHO even advised governments around the world to stock up on Tamiflu and Relenza well before the middle of 2009, when swine flu made its appearance.

Was it simply an incredible coincidence that pharmaceutical companies such as GlaxoSmithKline were prepared as early as 2008 to make vaccines against the 2009 H1N1 strain? In a media release dated May 15, 2009, the company said it was ready to go into production as soon as it received regulatory approval and that it had already received preliminary orders from several governments who intended to stock up on the vaccine in advance. How could the vaccine major have been so incredibly well-prepared a year in advance?

The UK had initially ordered 60 million doses, France 60 million doses, Belgium 12.6 million doses and Finland 5.3 million doses of H1N1 antigen, which the government would use along with its existing stocks of GlaxoSmithKline's adjuvant system.

The UK ended up buying a whopping 110 million doses of vaccine to immunize 80 percent of the population with two doses each! It eventually administered just 6 million doses or 5 percent of what it had ordered.

Not surprisingly, the world's richest nations are now trying to offload stocks and even cancel orders. The Netherlands, for instance, had placed an order for 19 million doses for sale to other countries, while Germany, which had ordered 50 million doses, is frantically trying to get vaccine-makers to cut that to half.

6. Money Wears A Mask

But while everyone was wondering about the pandemic that never was, some politicians were laughing all the way to the bank, among them former Defense Secretary Donald Rumsfeld.

An astute businessman and avowed friend of Big Pharma, Rumsfeld made a killing on the stock market in 2005 as the stock price of Tamiflu went through the roof after the 2004 WHO guidelines were released. Rumsfeld, who was chairman of Gilead Sciences from 1997 to 2001 (Gilead had developed Tamiflu and licensed it to Roche in 1996), owned at least $5 million of the stock, which leapt from $35 to $47 in April 2005.

Another US politician who made a killing is former Secretary of State George Shultz, who was on Gilead's board at the time. Shultz sold more than $7 million worth of the company's stock in 2005.

That wasn't the end of Tamiflu's honeymoon with the stock market. To create the illusion – actually, to push up their stock price further – Roche resorted to some pretty heavy-duty arm-twisting. The company announced in October 2005 that it would not manufacture any more Tamiflu unless the US government agreed to buy more of it. But then, panic buying took care of that. As the government picked up more Tamiflu, Roche backed down and got what it wanted anyway.

By the way, Rumsfeld's romance with Big Pharma goes much deeper. It was Rumsfeld who, as chairman of G D Searle, had persuaded the FDA to give the highly controversial artificial sweetener aspartame the thumbs-up. Used across the board in processed foods and as a 'sweetener for diabetics', aspartame is a carcinogenic agent and in extreme cases, can cause blindness and death.

But deadly side effects are not a concern for policy makers. An August 2009 study by Oxford researchers published in the BMJ raised questions about the wisdom of administering Tamiflu to children. This was based on a study which suggested that the cons outweighed the pros. At the crux of the study were complications in children who were administered the drug.

Still, the US government, in connivance with the FDA, needed to once again drum up demand for Tamiflu once the panic buying in 2005 had died down. Swine flu was the excuse. The reason: In 2006 alone, the US government had paid $20 million for 2 billion doses of Tamiflu and the stock was about to expire. While stirring up a media-generated storm, the government did something else. To protect itself, it changed the warning on the Tamiflu packet.

In 2006, the FDA warning read: "We are concerned that when/if the use of this drug increases in the US, there may be increasing cases of adverse consequence in the US." This warning followed several reports of delirium and suicide among children aged under 17 who were taking Tamiflu. Side effects occurred within a day or two and included panic attacks, delusions, convulsions, delirium, loss of consciousness, depression and in some cases suicide.

Post-swine flu, this warning was watered down to read: "People with the flu, particularly children, may be at an increased risk of self-injury and confusion shortly after taking Tamiflu and should be closely monitored for signs of unusual behavior." Magical, isn't it?

7. Pharma's Favorite Frontmen

I have repeatedly mentioned that the media does the bidding of Big Pharma. That's not new. Top-ranking executives in government office as well as politicians often make the switch to the boards of pharma companies including vaccine-makers and it is only when the link is exposed that one understands why the government makes certain decisions and how, say, a policy announcement, actually traces back to vaccine-makers and how that ultimately translates into big bucks for those involved.

But why sully the fair name of politicians only? The same unconscionable actions apply in equal measure to media moguls. Here are some stunning examples of just how the pharma-media-vaccine-dollars connection operates.

Remember the sudden 'shortage' of flu vaccines that surfaced in numerous media reports in October 2009? This 'shortage' can be traced back to a meeting held by an elite caucus of powerful and influential people who decide and direct global social, economic, financial, population and other policies – in anonymity.

In this instance, I am referring to a non-profit (how very ironic!) organization called the Council on Foreign Relations (CFR), whose puppeteers include media barons such as Rupert Murdoch (News Corp, Fox News, Associated Press, Twentieth Century Fox, Time Warner), Thomas Glocer (Reuters News Service) and Pulitzer Prize-winning journalist Laurie Garrett.

180

On October 16, 2009, the CFR's 'H1N1 Pandemic Study Group' met in New York. It was a meeting convened by Garrett, whose work is closely associated with the petrochemical-pharmaceutical cartel. The meeting was convened after sections of the public – those who did not buy into or were suspicious of the 'pandemic' lie – began to question the 'pandemic' that didn't pan out. Many began to question the need to get 'immunized' against swine flu and refused to take their shots.

As the public – and the Internet – became more vocal, vaccine manufacturers grew worried. Something had to be done. The media, a powerful influencing force of public opinion, had to be actively drawn into the act.

It is no coincidence that 'news' of a massive flu vaccine shortage surfaced a week after the CFR meeting. The idea was to ratchet up a shortage and make a public case for more vaccine sales. Declare the situation a national health emergency and the public will turn a blind eye to the fast-tracking of licenses that were so liberally handed out to GlaxoSmithKline, Novartis, CSL, Baxter, Sanofi Pasteur and others, to make a swine-flu vaccine.

But is it as simple as literally buying out media barons? Could the likes of Murdoch and Glocer be more directly linked to the flu vaccines? Well, here's an interesting nuance: Murdoch controls the Murdoch Children's Research Institute (MCRI) in Australia, which conducted the first H1N1 swine flu tests on children aged between 6 months and 8 years.

And another clue: Murdoch's son James is an overseer of GlaxoSmithKline's Board of Directors. The Murdoch connection doesn't end there. Rupert Murdoch's mother Elizabeth is a patron of the Royal Victoria Women's Hospital in Melbourne, Australia. The hospital's staff worked with CSL Pharmaceuticals to develop a swine flu vaccine.

Owned by Merck & Co, CSL is accused of testing their experimental swine flu vaccine on pregnant women without control subjects. Their safety tests lacked legitimate placebo controls and evaded long-term surveillance and data collection.

How about Thomas Glocer, CEO of Reuters? Glocer is also on the Board of Directors of Merck & Co and a member of the Partnership for New York City (PFNYC). Like the CFR, PFNYC is another caucus of powerful individuals who influence public policy, and whose primary beneficiaries are the drug industry. They do this by pushing the agenda for biotechnology and 'geneto-pharmaceuticals' across the world.

And guess who founded the PFNYC? None other than David Rockefeller, whose population agenda is familiar to readers of this book (See Chapter 3: Is There A Conspiracy?).

8. Storm In A Petri dish

There are allegations that the swine flu virus was manufactured in the laboratory alongside news that the CDC was creating a virus. Before we answer why a public health agency might want to do that, there are two key factors you must keep in mind. One, science still doesn't know enough about how viruses recombine and spread, and two, that coincidences in a combination of Big Pharma and public health agencies are usually no coincidence at all.

In a media statement dated November 24, 2009, the WHO had raised an odd but seemingly logical question: what if the deadly H5N1 avian flu virus of 2003 was to combine with the highly transmittable H1N1 virus that swept across continents in 2009?

The WHO claimed that new cases of avian flu had surfaced in Egypt, Indonesia and Vietnam in 2009, coinciding with the timeline that the swine flu virus was doing the rounds. Hence, the agency said there was cause to worry that the two types of viruses could produce a hybrid more deadly than H5N1 and more transmissible than N1N1.

Viruses are known to 'reassort', which is a process by which the genetic material from more than one virus mix in host cells to produce a new strain with features of the original strains. This was not the first time the WHO raised concerns over such a reassortment. The agency had raised the very same concerns in 2004, in the wake of the avian flu outbreak. Was this mere coincidence?

Also, oddly enough, exactly two months before the WHO spoke of a deadly hybrid in November 2009, the CDC was experimenting with just such a hybrid! Was it a coincidence?

Here are the facts. CDC scientists began experiments in the agency's labs where they injected ferrets with both the H1N1 virus and the lethal H5N1 avian flu virus in an attempt to see if they could 'reassort'. This was confirmed by Michael Shaw, the CDC's Associate Director for Laboratory Science for the agency's influenza division.

The avian flu virus was once thought to infect only poultry till it was observed to infect human beings in the 2003 outbreak that left around 500 people sick and killed more than 250 people. That's a 60 percent death rate. So it seemed that viruses thought to be confined to a single species could indeed jump species.

Next, the H1N1 virus, about which so little is still known, was observed to have infected turkeys in Chile. This supported the conclusion that this particular strain could transfer from human beings to birds.

Here is the next question: Was the swine flu virus genetically engineered? In other words, was it fabricated in a laboratory? It's a question that has spawned numerous conspiracy theories and the truth is there is no conclusive evidence yet.

But there are a couple of factors that lend credence to this supposition. One, pharma companies (remember Baxter's 'mix-up'?) and even the CDC, as mentioned above, have been playing with deadly viruses in their laboratories and these are only two instances that have come into public focus.

There is another reason why it is not difficult to believe that a lethal virus was deliberately unleashed. There are influential caucuses (remember Henry Kissinger?) who have declared that they aim to reduce the world's population by as much as 80 percent. And no matter how extreme that sounds, the fact is that powerful vested interests are always looking to control weaker nations with economics to secure control over their natural resources, among other things.

Crimes against humanity are all too familiar. Didn't the Nazis experiment with eugenics? Haven't the US and Israeli governments used bio-weapons before? Haven't global public health agencies used vaccines and mass immunization campaigns as vehicles to introduce viruses into Africa and other developing nations with devastating consequences?

The other reason to be suspicious is the hybrid nature of the 2009 strain of the H1N1 virus, which scientists say contains genetic material from strains of the North American bird flu, European swine flu, Asian swine flu and seasonal influenza viruses.

While it is not impossible for this hybrid to have evolved naturally, it is equally likely that it was genetically engineered. Governments along with major pharmaceutical companies have both the means and motive to do so.

That is precisely the way it appeared to have happened, and June 11, 2009, was a red-letter day – the day the WHO raised the outbreak to Level 6, that of a 'pandemic'. Of course, the WHO had neither hard evidence nor reason to take this decisive step, except to whip up global panic to the economic gain of vaccine-makers and their political minions.

What was the buildup to this critical decision? When in April, the swine flu outbreak seemed to be waning, senior representatives of vaccine majors met WHO Director-General Margaret Chan and United Nations Secretary General Ban Ki Moon at the WHO headquarters in Geneva in May 2009.

The ostensible reason was that this was to decide how to ship vaccines to developing nations. The secret agenda, on the other hand, was to justify raising the swine flu outbreak to a Level 6 pandemic. Once the Level 6 switch was thrown, vaccine-makers would make a killing!

When the outbreak began to decline, vaccine-makers panicked. Many of them had already signed deals with some developed nations to supply a 'pandemic vaccine' in the event of a, well, Level 6 pandemic. Germany, for instance, had signed just such a contract with GlaxoSmithKline in 2007.

Likewise, another overenthusiastic government was the UK government, whose key scientific advisor, Prof Roy Anderson, is also on GlaxoSmithKline's payroll. Anderson's annual payout by the vaccine maker is said to be $177,000.

GlaxoSmithKline had got to the German government as well. In June, a month before Level 6 was declared, the company asked the German government to confirm that they would indeed honor their contract to purchase the pandemic vaccine. When Big Pharma 'asks', it is never polite!

Thanks to some ground-breaking investigative work, and the grit and determination of many who seek the truth and nothing less than the truth about the swine flu outbreak, damning facts are continuing to emerge about the unholy nexus between the WHO, UN, developed countries and vaccine-makers who worked in unison to orchestrate the swine flu 'pandemic'.

9. Pandemic Fallout

Another question plaguing the plethora of vaccines unleashed on populations around the world is: Are they safe? If the answer is not obvious, then let me put it this way: The answer is a resounding 'no'!

There are many reasons why these vaccines should never enter the human body. At best, there is no proof that they are really effective. At worst, these synthetic chemical cocktails are alleged to have caused some of the deaths that took place during the 2009 outbreak.

But before we discuss that issue, here is another damning fact: All the vaccine-makers licensed to make the H1N1 vaccine were 'fast-tracked'. Simply put, the US FDA and its European counterpart, the European Medicines Agency (EMEA), hastily gave Big Pharma the green signal to manufacture vaccines that were not clinically tested.

Using the panic public health agencies so successfully whipped up as a cover, these agencies allowed vaccine manufacturers – GlaxoSmithKline, Novartis, Sanofi Pasteur, CSL, Medimmune and Baxter – to manufacture millions of doses which have been injected into populations across the globe without being sure of the consequences.

There have been no randomized, double-blind controlled placebo studies conducted on these vaccines and yet governments carried out mass immunization programs. But almost as soon as the chequered flag went up, complaints began to pour in.

Novartis's new swine flu vaccine Celtura, targeted at women and children, was rejected by the Swiss government due to concerns over its safety. There was suspicion that the vaccine manufacturer may have repackaged a 2008 vaccine, which had killed two dozen homeless people during an illegal clinical trial in Poland, and had passed it off as a vaccine against the new swine flu!

Another hazard is the recall of millions of doses by three vaccine majors shortly after they began supplying their drugs. Medimmune recalled just under 5 million doses of its nasal spray vaccine LAIV (Live Attenuated Influenza Vaccine) in December 2009 when it discovered that the vaccine's potency had declined. The US government had, by then, already ordered 40 million doses of LAIV.

In another monumental disaster, a week before the Medimmune debacle, Sanofi Pasteur recalled 800,000 pre-filled syringes of its swine flu monovalent vaccine when it discovered that doses meant for children had lost their potency.

Just a month before that, GlaxoSmithKline recalled their October batch of swine flu vaccine Pandemrix in Canada following reports of anaphylactic reactions in one out of 20,000 people who had been administered the drug. Anaphylactic reactions, which take place when the body goes into shock when foreign substances are introduced, can result in death.

Data with public health agencies is not easily available to public scrutiny but documents with the EMEA state that clinical trials conducted by GlaxoSmithKline on Pandemrix indicate that nervous system disorders were "very common" in those who had received it. Also "very common" were musculoskeletal and connective tissue disorders while blood and lymphatic system disorders were "common".

Canada was not the only country where Pandemrix met with stiff resistance. Switzerland too refused to buy the vaccine due to the serious side effects associated with it.

How do public health agencies, purportedly watchdogs of public health, give drugs like Pamdemrix the green signal? Here is how. Just like Novartis before it and Baxter later, GlaxoSmithKline had filed its patent for a 'pandemic flu vaccine', WO2006100109A1, on March 21, 2006. It then applied to the EMEA for permission to market its drug in February 2007.

This is an application for a very clever bit of jugglery authorized by the EMEA that helps fast-track vaccines when a pandemic actually breaks. It is called a 'mock-up' vaccine. The company received the go-ahead in May 2008, exactly a year before the swine flu 'pandemic' broke. How convenient!

But even more convenient is a 'mock-up vaccine' itself. According to the EMEA website, this is what it is. *"A mock-up pandemic influenza vaccine is a vaccine that mimics the future pandemic influenza vaccine in terms of its composition and manufacturing method. However, because the virus strain causing the pandemic is not known, the mock-up vaccine contains another flu strain instead. This is a strain that is not circulating in humans, and to which humans have not been exposed in the past. This enables the company to test its vaccine in preparation for any flu pandemic that may occur in the future, by carrying out studies with the mock-up vaccine that predict how people will react to the vaccine when the strain causing a pandemic is included."*

So when a pandemic or outbreak actually occurs, vaccine-makers merely switch the viral strain used in the mock-up vaccine for the one causing the outbreak and lo and behold! A new vaccine is approved and ready to be administered to millions of unsuspecting people.

In its application to the EMEA, GlaxoSmithKline offered the following facts about Pandemrix, which were actually reason enough to ban the vaccine. Instead, the company got the green signal.

"Safety pharmacology program: No safety pharmacology studies were performed with Pandemrix vaccine"

"Pharmacodynamic drug interactions: No studies were performed"
"Carcinogenicity: No carcinogenicity studies were conducted which is in line with the Note for Guidance on pre-clinical pharmacological and toxicological testing of vaccines"

Pandemrix was a cocktail for a medical catastrophe.

But it seems safety concerns over the drug went even deeper. According to an exposé by the British newspaper, *Daily Mail*, the UK government had reservations that Pandemrix may cause Guillain-Barré Syndrome (GBS), a sometimes-fatal nerve disease which could be triggered by the vaccine.

GBS, which results in respiratory distress and paralysis resulting from the degeneration of the myelin sheath covering the nerves, was conclusively linked to the vaccine involved in the 1976 swine flu debacle in the US (See Chapter 4: *Critical Mass*).

On July 29, 2009, Prof Elizabeth Miller, head of the UK's Health Protection Agency's Immunization Department, wrote a confidential letter to 600 senior neurologists asking them to look out for an increase in cases of GBS in individuals who had been vaccinated with Pandemrix. The letter specifically referred to the 1976 fiasco, where one person died of swine flu, 25 individuals died of GBS and at least 300 people were afflicted by the disease.

Prof Miller wrote in the letter: "It makes me feel wary that the government is rolling out this vaccine without any clear idea of the GBS risk, if any. I wouldn't wish it on anyone. I'm frightened to have the swine flu vaccine if this might happen again – it's a frightening illness and I think more research needs to be done on the effect of the vaccine."

Oddly enough, the confidential letter was sent to 600 neurologists in the UK but not to general practitioners who were liberally jabbing thousands of citizens with Pandemrix. Strangely, despite the government's public health agency raising these concerns, there was no investigation or inquiry launched into the vaccine.

There is no doubt that the swine flu vaccines being sold across the world are dangerous, even lethal, cocktails of untested chemicals containing viral genetic material. Yet at the height of the 'pandemic', the US government stated that children and pregnant women would be at the frontlines of those who should receive these drugs.

Schools always provide a captive population for pharma companies – where else do you get so many innocent and willing victims all in one place to test? – and the swine flu outbreak of 2009 was no exception. So as children lined up, not knowing what fate awaited them, they innocently lent their bodies to unscrupulous vaccine-makers who turned schools into testing centers.

Not surprisingly, pregnant women who had been vaccinated against swine flu began to report miscarriages soon after they took their shots.

Has the CDC been lying about the safety of vaccines, and continues to do so? In September 2010, the National Coalition of Organized Women (NCOW) presented data from two different sources demonstrating that the 2009/10 H1N1 vaccines contributed to as many as 3,587 cases of miscarriage and still deaths. Although the CDC knew of the data, it continued to assure pregnant women, a prime vaccine target group, and vaccine providers that the vaccine posed no risk for pregnant women.

The two sources comprised data from NCOW's own survey covering pregnant women aged 17-45 and the Vaccine Adverse Event Reporting System (VAERS). Needless to say, during the Advisory Commission on Childhood Vaccines (ACCV) meeting on September 3, 2010, Eileen Dannemann, Director of NCOW, informed Dr Marie McCormick, Chairperson of the CDC's Vaccine Risk and Assessment Working Group about these shocking findings for a second time. With full knowledge of the NCOW data then publically available, Dr McCormick stated there were absolutely no H1N1 vaccine-related adverse events in pregnant women in 2009/10.

Based on the assessment group's baseless and erroneous announcement that these vaccines are perfectly safe for pregnant women, the CDC's Advisory Committee on Immunization Practices (ACIP) has issued the recommendation to give the 2010/11 flu to all people, including pregnant women. In her report, Dannemann noted that the upcoming 2010/11 flu vaccine contains the same elements that are implicated in the killing of these fetuses, the H1N1 viral component and the neurotoxin mercury (Thimerosal) plus two other viral strains.

On a third occasion, during the September 14, 2010 National Vaccine Advisory Committee (NVAC) meeting, Dannemann submitted the data for the third time during public comment and asked: "Why hasn't Dr. McCormick looked in the VAERS database?"

The NCOW report states: "It must be argued that the CDC was grossly negligent to fail to inform their vaccine providers of the incoming VAERS data, while providers blindly followed the CDC 'standard of care' guidelines to vaccinate every pregnant woman in 2009/10. Furthermore, in the face of these findings and the purposeful withholding of these findings by CDC's Dr Marie McCormick and her vaccine risk assessment group, for the CDC's Advisory Committee on Immunization Practices (ACIP) to recommend another iteration of the same vaccine to pregnant women in 2010/11 may be argued as more than gross negligence - but rather - an act of willful misconduct."

In spite of the damning evidence of irreparable harm done by vaccinating pregnant women, as of today, there is no indication that the CDC and its assessment group are considering to back down from their position.

The NCOW is now left with no other choice than to recommend that the CDC at least adheres to the FDA/manufacturers warning on the vaccine's insert package which states that the flu shot should not be given to pregnant women unless clearly needed. NCOW publically requested the CDC to "advise all Ob/Gyns, vaccine providers and the public this year, of last season's VAERS reports on H1N1 vaccine-related fetal deaths". However, it is unlikely for the CDC to follow the NCOW's recommendations as these would expose its fraudulent stance.

Children and pregnant women, both extremely vulnerable sections of the population, were deliberately targeted even as vaccine-makers admitted to having no safety data to explain this barbaric step. Moreover, governments in many developed nations did nothing to warn their citizens of these dangers. But why would they? Read on.

10. On The Fast Track

What happens when vaccines and other drugs are fast-tracked? We have just discussed 'mock-up' vaccines and the utter lack of clinical testing. In the late 1990s and early 2000s, around two dozen drugs for cancer were fast-tracked for approval by the FDA. Thousands of cancer patients received these experimental drugs, especially terminal patients.

How can one assess the efficacy of these drugs when they were tested only on a minuscule sample in an attempt to apply for hasty approval? Also, the toxicity of a drug – a critical parameter assessed during approval – can only be evaluated after a certain amount of time has elapsed. Fast-tracking a drug therefore doesn't take into account the long-term side effects it could have.

In a study by Northwestern University Medical School, it was found that cancer drugs Velcade had been tested on only 188 subjects, Mylotarg on 142, Campath on 93 and Clolar on 49 subjects before they were approved!

Administering experimental drugs to terminal patients and justifying it by saying the benefits might outweigh the downside is tantamount to using these patients as human guinea pigs.

In the words of Patricia Keegan, Director of the FDA's division of Therapeutic Biological Oncology Products, cancer drugs need to be administered in high doses to be effective. "Finding a completely safe drug is probably not an achievable goal. It's really more a question of balancing," she said.

One would think that when drugs are fast-tracked, the FDA would insist that drug makers conduct long-term follow-up studies to assess the drugs' safety. Though this is a requirement on paper, it is usually not enforced. There isn't a single case of a fast-tracked drug being recalled for want of a follow-up study.

The Vioxx debacle (See Chapter 5: *The Vaccine Hangover*) is a glaring example of what happens when the FDA turns a blind eye to lack of rigorous testing. The pain-reliever recommended for arthritic patients caused 38,000 serious cases of cardiac arrest and death and was eventually recalled in 2004.

This Merck drug was reintroduced in the market a year later after a panel of 32 experts voted to bring it back on the market. It later transpired that 10 of the 32 advisers on the FDA panel, which had also voted in favor of controversial drugs Celebrex and Bextra, had strong financial links to the companies that made these drugs – Pfizer and Novartis respectively.

It is disheartening, to say the least, that Big Pharma should enjoy complete immunity to crimes that jeopardize human lives, and that the FDA and CDC should so brazenly give drug makers free rein to continue their malpractices. It is therefore in the interest of your health that you seriously stop to ask yourself if there isn't a better way to achieve good health than allowing yourself to fall prey to the deceitful promises made by pharmaceutical companies.

While on the subject of lack of testing, the H1N1 vaccine too is an untested vaccine and no drug manufacturer can say that is clinically proven to be safe. Not surprisingly, after the H1N1 vaccine was introduced into the population, an avalanche of adverse reactions was reported from various countries.

For instance, the province of British Columbia in Canada recorded double the number of severe allergic reactions and cases of anaphylactic shock. Residents here had received Arepanrix, which had been authorized despite lack of clinical testing. Some doctors believed the unusually large number of cases with serious side effects was because some people had received the swine flu vaccine along with the seasonal flu shot. Either way, the reaction was due to vaccination.

In another Canadian province, Manitoba, GlaxoSmithKline's Arepanrix was pulled out after doctors were alarmed over the number of "life-threatening reactions" post-vaccination.

The vaccine was triggering so many anaphylactic reactions that more than 170,000 doses of one batch had to be benched. Though the authorities tried to water down the incident, the fact is that 36 severe adverse events were recorded. These included severe allergic reactions within minutes of receiving the H1N1 shot. Tucked away among this statistics was one fatality.

Take a look at the shocking guidelines on the package insert of Arepanrix and you will not be surprised. The guidelines admit that "there is no clinical experience for this vaccine or its comparison, H5N1, in the elderly, children or adolescents". The trials they have data on are only for healthy adults aged 18-60!

If that isn't contradictory, get this. The company admits that it has no data on pregnant or breastfeeding women, either. Yet, governments across the globe had been coaxing and coercing children and pregnant women to get vaccinated with Arepanrix.

According to the vaccine maker, the clinical trials to collect data on Arepanrix were taking place as "the current injections are being given". It doesn't take much to read between the lines. In other words, the mass vaccination drives using this drug were precisely the experiments the company needed to test the drug. The government had allowed the company access to millions of gullible human guinea pigs!

And yes, the pharma industry even has a term for it – "post-marketing surveillance", where a drug maker is allowed to submit data on the safety and effectiveness of the drug as it is administered as a test drug.

Canada was not the only country to notice that the vaccine was causing anaphylactic reactions in vaccinated individuals. In November 2009, the Turkish Republic released a memorandum to its vaccine centers, asking them to keep an eye open for "frightening side effects" to this vaccine. The memorandum was apparently sent after a doctor went into a coma after his H1N1 shot.

Meanwhile, in Sweden, there were five reported fatalities and 350 reports of adverse events immediately after people were vaccinated with the highly controversial Pandemrix. Separately, in a Swedish school, 130 students reported sick after a vaccination drive the previous day. In some countries, deaths were reported within hours of being vaccinated for swine flu.

Seizures, persistent nausea and vomiting were the least of the complaints received by doctors. Many reports from across countries included GBS-like symptoms and paralysis.

Remember Jordan McFarland, the 14-year-old from Virginia in the US, whose picture was splashed across the media being wheeled out of hospital after receiving his H1N1 shot? The teenager was reportedly afflicted with GBS-like symptoms within hours of receiving the vaccine.

There were also reports of deaths in Sweden, Japan and China. According to these reports, some people had died only hours after receiving the swine flu vaccine. Among the deceased was a Chinese teacher. The government immediately shelved the batch of vaccines from which the suspect dose was administered.

Amid the deluge of reports of adverse reactions in China, a Chinese newspaper reported more than 1,200 cases of side effects ranging from sore arms, rashes and headaches to anaphylactic shock and sudden drops in blood pressure.

11. The S-Word

Finally, there's the S-word – squalene. This is a natural substance present in the body found throughout the brain and nervous system. Squalene is a healthy substance that has antioxidant properties when it is naturally present. It is an oily substance that is also present in olive oil and safflower oil and studies have linked squalene to a reduction in the risk of cancer.

So far so good. Now when vaccine-makers Novartis and GlaxoSmithKline decided to introduce squalene into their H1N1 vaccines, it kicked up a furor among sections of the medical community. When this oil-based chemical is used in a vaccine, it is called an adjuvant, whose sole purpose is to turbo-charge the drug.

This means, squalene boosts or exaggerates the immune response to the vaccine to make it 'more effective'. The other reason why squalene is used in vaccines is so that more of the antigen (the inactivated or weakened/attenuated virus used in the vaccine) can go around. More potent vaccines mean less of the antigen needs to be used in each dose. More antigen available means more vaccines and more vaccines means no shortages and therefore more money in the bank for Big Pharma.

But why should something that reduces the risk of cancer be harmful – even potentially lethal – when introduced into a vaccine? The answer lies in the route through which it is administered. When injected (as opposed to being eaten in foods and therefore being naturally introduced), the body perceives squalene as an enemy and begins to attack it. The problem is the body then begins to perceive all squalene, irrespective of its origins, as an enemy.

The immune system proceeds to attack and destroy the substance wherever it finds it in the body, which is effectively an autoimmune response. This is why squalene and some other substances in vaccines are associated with autoimmune disorders such as GBS.

Squalene is the culprit that is now conclusively linked to the devastating autoimmune disorders suffered by thousands of Gulf War veterans who were involved in Operation Desert Shield and Desert Storm in the Persian Gulf. US soldiers received the adjuvant in the anthrax vaccines they were forcibly administered.

Novartis (M59) and GlaxoSmithKline (ASO3) are two drug companies that use squalene in their swine flu vaccines. Though cleared for use in Europe, the dangerous adjuvant was not given the green signal in the US, thanks to a vigilant public. But there is cause for concern for US citizens: The US government bought the adjuvant worth more than a billion dollars to stock up just in case it needed to invoke its Emergency Use Authorization (EUA). In other words, the US government is sitting on a lethal bio-time bomb.

Even if one believes that squalene has not yet been used in vaccines in the US, the fact remains that millions of people in Europe have received this dangerous substance. During those assembly line-like mass vaccination drives during the swine flu 'pandemic', there is no way of telling just how many hundreds and thousands of children and young adults are now at risk of developing autoimmune disorders.

If you think that the swine flu is now history and we can all move on, think again, especially if you consider getting a seasonal flu shot. Although there is no indication that we will have another swine flu epidemic any time soon, the untested H1N1 swine flu vaccine is being included in the annual flu jab this winter (2010-2011).

This makes a lot of sense, given the necessity to reduce the enormous stocks of the vaccine that governments were lured into ordering last year. The groups targeted during the new vaccination campaign are also the ones who will experience the most side effects, namely the elderly, children, and those suffering from such conditions as heart disease, respiratory ailments and diabetes.

Of course, it makes no difference to health policy makers that a new study published in the Journal of American Medical Association provides evidence that the 2009 H1N1 flu virus had a significantly lower risk of causing serious complications than found during other recent influenza outbreaks. According to the study by Edward A. Belongia, M.D. and colleagues, the 2009 H1N1 flu did not increase hospitalizations and cases of pneumonia.

Instead of advising the public on how to prevent getting the flu through well-researched and time-tested immune-building approaches, health protection agencies merely call on everyone to receive their annual toxin-filled flu shot. Natural immune-builders includes restoring depleted vitamin D levels through regular sun exposure without sun protection, taking oleander extract, Echinacea, Pau d'arco, Suma, Astragalus, medicinal mushrooms, Beta glucans, Aloe vera, Colloidal Silver, olive leaf extract, oil of wild mountain oregano, turmeric, black seed oil (Nigella sativa), Master Mineral Supplement (MMS), or grapefruit seed extract. (I have discussed this further in Chapter 9: The Whole Truth)

Chapter 8

A-tishoo! Of Lies

Before discussing seasonal influenza per se, let us return to the premise that 'germs cause disease'. Starting with Louis Pasteur, who propounded this germ theory in the 19th century, to Western medicine, we have been led to believe that pathogens – all manner of microbes including bacteria and viruses – are waiting to attack us and make us ill.

The second assumption is that the presence of a virus in the human body implies that the individual has contracted a disease specific to that virus. Painting a picture of 'deadly viruses' is pure medieval thinking. It is incorrect to assume that when a virus (rather, antibodies to a presumed virus) is present in a person who died of a disease that the virus killed him/her.

And it is not just the presence of a virus that seems to suggest that an individual is infected. Here is an eye-opener. Did you know that HIV tests do not test for the HIV virus but the presence of antibodies to the virus? Antibodies are present to fend off disease, or heal a person, and their mere presence in the body does not mean that the individual has contracted the disease. Yet when an HIV test detects the presence of antibodies, the individual is labeled as being infected with the HIV virus. However, this is actually what medicine calls a false positive (it seems to be HIV, but isn't).

In my book, *Ending the AIDS myth*, I cite research that shows close to 95 percent of HIV diagnosis is false positive, ruining and wrecking the lives of these diagnosed individuals.

Also, people who are vaccinated against the HIV virus will invariably end up testing positive on subsequent HIV tests as vaccines are designed to make the body produce antibodies against the virus.

This is a clever trick employed by diagnostic facilities and pharmaceutical companies, who benefit considerably as HIV patients are usually administered expensive, life-long medication. Smart thinking, isn't it?

Also, when doctors detect the virus in the body of an AIDS victim, they conclude that the patient died of AIDS. But there are now dozens of AIDS diseases, which are basically combinations of conditions like pneumonia or African wasting disorder and specific antibodies to a presumed virus (HIV).

A person who dies from pneumonia with a positive HIV test is automatically presumed to have died from AIDS although it has never been proved that HIV can cause AIDS. And to reiterate, even Dr Luc Antoine Montagnier, the main discoverer of the Human Immunodeficiency Virus, says that HIV alone cannot cause AIDS. He says HIV is harmless and doesn't need to be treated and that the focus should be on hygiene, clean water and nutrition.

The point I am making is that viruses are present in our body for a reason. There are many of them present – even some of the 'deadly' ones – at all times without us even knowing it. And they are present for us to perform specific functions – these inert protein fragments help the body heal just like bacteria and fungi help the body break down or decompose damaged or dead cells.

When the body is damaged and weak, these germs get activated and help the body heal in many different ways. They begin to feed on dead cells and debris; they help in the manufacture of chemicals to compensate for deficient processes and, as in the case of cancer, grow extra cells to 'make up' for damaged tissues.

Viruses often act as solvents that dissolve harmful chemicals and even toxic heavy metals and other pollutants. The more toxins we have in our body, the more likely will the body facilitate the production of such proteins. Hence, disease is a sign that toxic processes have risen beyond the body's ability to handle them.

Also, being inert protein particles, viruses have no reproductive capabilities. They require a host to reproduce. The host is the human body or an animal. The human body is highly intelligent and it has no biological program that causes it to attempt suicide. If it reproduces such protein fragments ('viruses'), it does this for a reason. To call them 'deadly viruses' is farfetched, to say the least.

Thus, when an individual takes ill, it is not the virus that has made him/her ill. The causes of disease lie elsewhere. Viruses and bacteria are simply trying to help. The symptoms that result from their activity are nothing but a signal that the body is trying to heal itself.

Here is an analogy. If an apple falls from a tree and is bruised or damaged, would an intelligent person claim that the apple is being infected and killed by deadly bacteria? The answer is no, because it is common sense that bacteria naturally decompose the damaged part of the apple because it no longer serves a purpose, that is, a source of food.

Likewise, if a number of cells in our body are damaged due to internal congestion, poor oxygenation, Vitamin D deficiency due to lack of sun exposure, irregular sleep habits, consuming immune-suppressive junk food, it is completely natural for similar cell-specific germs to enter our body, and further damage and decompose these already damaged, weak cells because they are no longer useful.

When a person succumbs to an ever-increasing influx of poisons (through food, air, water, drugs, etc), we can also expect to find an excessive presence of these protein fragments, falsely called viruses, during an autopsy. If a pet dies and its owner has multiple sclerosis or chronic fatigue syndrome, shouldn't we first ask what type of toxins both of them were exposed to that caused the body to take recourse to such extreme defense mechanisms as mass-producing protein fragments needed to combat these toxins? Did both of them breathe the same pollution-filled air produced by heavy traffic on a busy street or by a chemical factory nearby?

Of course, an autopsy will find the presence of large amounts of specific antibodies to such specific toxins in the blood of the diseased animal and its owner. Blaming an inert, lifeless virus for killing them is unscientific, misleading and irresponsible, and spreading fear about an imminent and deadly viral epidemic should be left to those who make a living out of deluding the masses.

Fear suppresses the immune system. That is a fact. I question the intentions of anyone who purposely spreads such misinformation, under the pretense of wanting to protect us, when panic does nobody any good.

1. Winter's Cold, Dark Secret

Having said that, let us focus our attention on seasonal flu and the myths that cause millions of people to run scared with the approach of winter, especially in the cold, temperate regions. For people who live in these countries, not taking the annual 'flu shot' is associated with fear and is viewed as an invitation to imminent illness, even death. Twisting nature to suit their own objectives, vaccine-makers have hit upon a clever way to make pots of profits.

But first, let us talk about why people get the flu. The clue to that answer is precisely the time of year – winter – when the flu breaks out. Contrary to popular belief, it is not dropping temperatures but the lack of sufficient sunlight exposure that is responsible for the flu choosing to surface during these bleak months.

The seasonal flu virus spreads in the human body because the body's immune system is weak – and not because it is cold. In turn, the body is weak during this time due to low Vitamin D levels as sunlight is weak and people tend to stay indoors during the fall and winter months.

Think about it. Flu outbreaks do not take place in summer when Vitamin D production in the body increases (in healthy response to sun exposure). A weak immune system cannot keep the body clean, and a bacterial or viral infection becomes necessary to cleanse it. This natural response to an unnatural situation is not a disease and should be supported, not suppressed.

Vitamin D is crucial to staying healthy. Though usually associated with calcium absorption and bone health, it plays a vital role in two other important bodily processes – immunity, and gene transcription and expression.

In a study conducted at Jikei University School of Medicine Minato-ku in Tokyo, researchers found that Vitamin D was 8 percent more effective in preventing the flu in children compared to those who were not exposed to Vitamin D supplements. But when compared to children who are vaccinated, these supplements were 800 percent more effective.

This study is one among many that support greater sunlight exposure for enhanced immunity. But first, Vitamin D needs to be activated in the body and the best way to do this is, again, by getting enough sunlight. That is, by allowing your skin to be exposed to the healing ultraviolet band in sunlight.

When UV light falls on the skin, it kick-starts a process whereby Vitamin D is converted into its active form in the liver and kidneys. But recent research by the University of Iowa published in the *Journal of Immunology* has found that Vitamin D can be activated in pulmonary cells as well, specifically in the airways.

Researchers found a connection between Vitamin D produced in the airways of the lungs and the activation of two genes that help prevent infection. While one gene expresses a protein called cathelicidin that can kill bacteria, the second gene produces a protein that helps cells recognize other types of pathogens.

Interestingly, other organs that were found to express the enzyme that converts Vitamin D into its active form are the intestines, breast and prostate. In an interesting finding, the research team also observed that some of the Vitamin D acted locally. That is, while active Vitamin D produced by the kidneys circulates in the bloodstream, Vitamin D converted by the other organs does not circulate and protect these organs from infection.

The study also stressed the role of Vitamin D in controlling inflammation, which when prolonged, contributes to autoimmune diseases such as multiple sclerosis and Type 1 diabetes as well as some cancers.

There is a vast body of research which has demonstrated that sufficient amounts of Vitamin D protect against influenza and other upper respiratory tract illnesses and is linked to the production of an anti-bacterial peptide called cathelicidin. But this peptide does more than that. Cathelicidin is a signaling molecule in the immune system and plays a significant role in the body's general immunity.

Some studies on Vitamin D have found that the vitamin dampens the effect of TNFa, which is an inflammatory cytokine. These cytokines are essential when the body is trying to stave off an infection. But if TNFa levels are already consistently high (as in the case of obesity, asthma and arthritis and autoimmune disorders), Vitamin D will lower the body's TNFa levels. Hence, when there is a need to elevate it, as is the case during a viral infection, the body will do so naturally.

The benefits of Vitamin D cannot be overstated. Japanese scientists, who published their findings in the *American Journal of Clinical Nutrition*, found that while anti-viral drugs zanamivir and oseltamivir bring down the risk of flu in children by 8 percent, exposure to Vitamin D brings it down by 50 percent.

Getting sufficient amounts of Vitamin D though sunlight exposure and supplements also means stronger bones and teeth, a well-regulated immune system, and a reduced risk of heart disease, autoimmune disorders and cancer. Moreover, sun-induced Vitamin D has no side effects. The same cannot be said for vaccines.

2. The Flu Is Not Passed On

What amazes me is that there is this almost unshakeable notion that the flu can be passed on from person to person, although studies have clearly shown that infection does not occur in every person who is exposed to the same virus. Typically, only 10 percent or fewer subjects exposed to a virus develop symptoms. In those 10 percent, the body uses the virus to mop up accumulated noxious substances.

In the rest, the body is capable of doing this without the help of such a solvent.

Many people live in complete isolation but still develop the seasonal flu because their body makes a strain of virus that is most conducive to cleansing itself of toxins. That is also why the seasonal flu virus mutates from one season to another. This is essential for the human body's survival. If there were just one type of flu virus, the body would develop immunity and never get the opportunity to purge itself of toxins, if this becomes necessary.

Now every year, the CDC says that 36,000 Americans die from the flu. And it uses this 'statistic' to scare the public into taking their annual flu shot. Have you ever wondered why this figure doesn't change, not even by a single digit, year after year?

The truth is, as admitted by the CDC on its own website, the 36,000 figure was picked from a 2003 study published in the Journal of the American Medication Association. This study had analyzed data from flu seasons all through the 1990s. It had looked at death certificates which cited the cause of death as 'respiratory or circulatory disease' and used 'statistical modeling' and arrived at 36,000 flu deaths!

This is pure guesswork and is odd, considering that when government health agencies want to play down a disease, they harp on lab-confirmed results. Why not for a figure publicly read on its website? Moreover, the CDC has made no attempt to repeat this guesswork (to update the figure) for close to a decade! Could this have anything to do with the fact that 'influenza' is rarely listed as cause of death on death certificates?

Another fact that public health agencies fail to take into account is that in many elderly people (the incidence of influenza is higher in children and the elderly than other age groups) who succumb to multiple illnesses, influenza is usually a secondary complication. Merely contracting the flu cannot hold the virus responsible for death.

But the CDC is very adept at throwing alarming figures at the American public. The problem is, it is way off the mark most of the time. Dr Tom Jefferson, head of vaccine studies at the prestigious international Cochrane Database Collaboration, points to some interesting CDC predictions of influenza strains gone wrong!

After performing his own statistical analysis, he found that for the 1992-1993 influenza season, the CDC was wrong by 84 percent; for the 1994-1995 season, 43 percent for the primary strain and 87 percent and 76 percent for two other strains; and for the 1997-1998 season, 84 percent.

However, what we do know is this: 61,777 people die from pneumonia every year in the US (2001 deaths: Final data for 2001, NCHS, CDC). Pneumonia is caused by severe respiratory congestion that requires bacteria to intervene. Yet bacteria are blamed for causing the illness. Still, public health agencies tend to confuse pneumonia with the flu, further muddying the flu debate.

In most cases, pneumonia is treated with antibiotics, which prevent lung detoxification. The antibiotics further suppress the natural defenses of the body, thereby preventing it from mopping up the drug chemicals. When a flu infection occurs, and the patient dies from respiratory failure in spite of it, the doctor may be tempted to say it was the flu that killed the patient. In truth, however, the patient died from internal congestion and a weak immune system.

Young children whose immune systems have been severely compromised by vaccines, and the elderly who are on at least two to three prescription drugs which always act as immune-suppressants, and who receive regular flu shots, are the most susceptible to developing flu symptoms.

Keeping the immune system strong and the body clean through liver, colon and kidney cleanses (See my book The Amazing Liver and Gallbladder Flush for details) is the best we can do to get through these trying times of increasing contamination. Also include avoiding doctors, hospitals, surgeries, drugs and vaccines, as well as getting enough sleep (eight to nine hours every night), eating fresh, nutritious food, avoiding processed foods and animal proteins, and getting sufficient sun exposure to keep vitamin D levels up.

3. Flu Vaccines Don't Work

Vaccines have never been shown to be more effective than doing nothing at all. Quite the contrary, they have contributed to numerous outbreaks of diseases, which I have discussed in great detail in my book Timeless Secrets of Health and Rejuvenation.

For example, in 1918-19, during the Spanish avian flu outbreak, only those soldiers and other people who were vaccinated against the flu actually fell ill and died, often right after receiving the shots. Millions of people died of the lethal vaccines to which the body had no natural defenses. Those who refused the vaccine remained healthy, in spite of helping the sick and carrying away the dead.

The vaccine industry insists that their vaccines against the flu serve as the key to a healthy winter. That is why in many countries with a severe winter, there's a headlong scramble by the public to get their annual flu shot.

Influenza always starts in the Far East and then spreads to the West in early winter, reaching its peak during February and March. It may come in either of three types, A, B, or C. During the last several years, Type A has been the dominant active strain. What makes vaccination against the flu so unsuccessful is that the flu virus mutates very quickly and there is a new one active every year. Also, the so-called protection offered by vaccines lasts for only six months. So every autumn, you require a new vaccination for a different virus. The trouble is, drug companies have no way of knowing in the summer which new strain of the flu virus is going to strike in the Western Hemisphere during the winter months. Accordingly, millions of people get vaccinated against an old, outdated strain for nothing, except to develop a weaker immune system and develop other side effects which may include flu symptoms.

Although a serious flu epidemic has not occurred for almost 40 years, their vaccines are prescribed to millions of people each year. You may wonder why perfectly healthy people are injected with a normally harmless bug whose strains mutate from year to year. While flu vaccines can never be accurate, employers encourage millions of their employees to submit to a flu shot each year, trying to avoid the loss of working days.

Studies on the so-called efficacy of the seasonal flu vaccine have repeatedly shown that the 'flu shot' has little bearing on the incidence of the disease. But nothing stirred the debate as did the results of a new study led by Canadian researchers who demonstrated that vaccinating health workers who work in homes for the elderly had no effect whatsoever on the incidence of flu in their wards.

The conclusions were based on five studies conducted between 1997 and 2009. According to Dr Roger Thomas of the University of Calgary, lead author of the paper published by the Cochrane Library, and Dr Tom Jefferson, the paper's co-author and vaccine expert with the Cochrane Database Collaboration, the study showed that immunizing health workers had no effect on laboratory-confirmed influenza; it did not bring down the incidence of pneumonia among the senior citizens; and it had no bearing on the death rate from pneumonia in the target group.

As for vaccinating the elderly themselves, studies whose findings have been published in the American Journal of Respiratory and Critical Care Medicine indicate that deaths from influenza and pneumonia in senior citizens remain unchanged even though vaccination has gone up from 15 percent in 1980 to 65 percent at present in this age group.

The Japanese authorities, for their part, have been more honest after research in that country proved that flu shots were a waste of public money. Japan had implemented compulsory flu vaccination for school children during the 1980s. However, after two large studies, which included children from four cities and varying vaccination rates, showed that the shots did not impact on the seasonal flu, mandatory immunization was stopped in 1987. In fact, two years later, it was found that only 20 percent of the general population elected to take the seasonal influenza vaccine.

Many vaccine producers grow the vaccines, consisting of live viruses, in hen's eggs. When the vaccine is injected into the body, it can cause side effects such as redness and soreness at the injection site and a mild form of flu. Very serious complications arise in people who are taking immune-suppressing drugs or who have a heart condition. If you are allergic to eggs, a flu-shot may also endanger your health. Of course, if a person with a pre-existing heart or lung condition dies after receiving a flu shot, doctors will blame the condition for his death, and not the flu vaccine.

For the average healthy person, coming down with the flu is not serious at all. On the contrary, it can build up natural immunity even against future encounters with new strains of the flu virus. The very reason that nature creates these new forms of virus every year and spreads them with accurate timing is to ensure continued ecological balance and strong immunity in plants, animals, and humans alike. However, it is rare for a person whose vitamin D levels remain optimal and whose liver and gallbladder are clean to get the flu.

Anyone prone to repeated infections is likely to have a toxic liver with many hundreds of stones accumulated in the liver and gallbladder. Gallstones, which harbor many types of infectious bacteria and viruses, are a constant source of immune suppression. Cleansing the liver and gallbladder of all gallstones (including intrahepatic gallstones found in the liver and calcified gallstones found in the gallbladder) offers about the best protection against any type of infection. People who have cleansed their liver in this way have reported that they never catch a cold or the flu any more.

Flu virus vaccines used until 2002 contained 'live' viruses and produced so many serious, adverse reactions that new vaccines had to be concocted. The new formula for flu vaccines is called the 'subvirion', which basically is a mutilated virus 'blended, spliced and macerated' until just bits and pieces of the original virus are left. This in no way makes the virus less dangerous. In fact, the antigens or foreign proteins in the vaccine, for which the body is forced to produce antibodies, are still as poisonous and harmful as the live virus.

Besides the subvirion, plenty of other substances are added to the flu vaccine, most of which you would never want to consciously ingest. These include:

- Hemagglutinin antigens that cause clumping of the red blood cells, leading to cardiovascular disease.
- The enzyme neuraminidase, which cuts out neuraminic acid from the cell membrane, weakening the trillions of cell membranes in the body.
- A white crystalline substance called allantoin, a toxic animal waste product. Due to its high nitrogen content, allantoin is used as fertilizer; it leads to kidney and bladder stones in humans.
- Gentamicin, a broad spectrum antibiotic, is added to each embryonated chicken egg to inhibit the growth of bacteria (vaccine is grown in chicken eggs).
- Formaldehyde (carcinogenic), used as a preservative and to inactivate the virus.
- The toxic chemicals, tri butylphosphate and Polysorbate 80, U.S.P.
- Resin, to eliminate "substantial portions" of tri butylphosphate and Polysorbate 80
- Thimerosal, a mercury derivative, to preserve the vaccine cocktail.
- Polyethylene glycol, a relative of ethylene glycol (antifreeze); often used to poison dogs and other predators of sheep.
- Isocctylphenyl ether, a compound of ether; has anesthetic properties; a teratogen, causing abnormal prenatal development. It also induces testicular atrophy in animals.

Vaccine producers are unable to guarantee that the vaccine will protect you against the flu. So they carefully tell you that the vaccine "reduces the likelihood of infection; or if you do develop the disease, it will be a milder case". Some express the same uncertainty about their product in this way: "It is known definitely that influenza virus vaccine, as now constituted, is not effective against all possible strains of influenza virus." Perhaps the best lesson of this effect comes from Japan. Compulsory flu vaccination in Japan (1967-1987) revealed no benefit and actually caused more flu- and vaccine-related deaths.

Why would you want to entrust your health to a cocktail of poisonous chemicals when even a somewhat weakened immune system stands a far better chance of protecting you against harm from a bout of influenza? Our body's sophisticated immune system, which has evolved over millions of years, can certainly do a better job of protecting you against the flu than anything manmade.

All it needs is some basic caretaking on your part. With each new flu shot, on the other hand, your immune system becomes more depleted and the side effects become more pronounced and severe. And, you may still get the flu anyway. The following list includes the possible consequences you might develop if you choose to go down the vaccination path:

The most frequent side effects of vaccination:

- Soreness at the site of the vaccination
- Pain or tenderness
- Erythema
- Inflammation
- Skin discoloration
- Induration
- A mass or lump
- Hypersensitivity reactions including puritus and urticaria
- Fever
- Malaise
- Myalgia
- Arthralgia
- Asthenia
- Chills
- Dizziness

- Headache
- Lymphadenopathy
- Rash
- Nausea
- Vomiting
- Diarrhea
- Pharyngitis
- Angiopathy
- Vasculiltis
- Anaphylaxis in asthmatics, with possible death
- Anaphylactic shock, with possible death

4. Flu Vaccine Conspiracy?

Vaccination certainly does not create immunity. You cannot become immune by ingesting poisons that destroy the immune system. Studies by a group of Italian scientists showed that the flu vaccine reduced the occurrence of clinical episodes of influenza by only 6 percent in adults, and effectiveness tended to decrease with age. They concluded that universal immunization wasn't warranted.

Stated simply, hand-washing and other hygienic and nutritional measures are far superior to the flu vaccine. If you practice good hygiene, eat nutritious foods and keep your intestines and liver clean, influenza will never become a deadly disease. Getting vaccinated against the flu, on the other hand, is a sure way to sow the seeds for new illnesses in the body. All vaccines are poisonous and, as such, act like time bombs that will explode in due time.

Now here is something that will make you sit up and take notice. It goes by the codename: 'US patent No 5911998 – Method of producing a virus vaccine from an African green monkey kidney cell line'. Now many are aware that viruses are grown in the organs of animals, which is dangerous enough (See Chapter 2: *Historical Blunders and the SV40 virus*) but what's really intriguing is the entity that owns this patent.

The owner is Dyncorp, a private military contractor working with the US government. Dyncorp's tagline on its website says the company aims "to make the world a safer place". The company, listed on the New York Stock Exchange, describes itself as "a global government services provider in support of US national security and foreign policy objectives..."

Dyncorp claims it helps make the world a safer place. Yet, the company is accused of human rights violations and genocide in Bosnia, Ecuador and Columbia. Its services were also hired by the US government to patrol the US-Mexico border, where the swine flu virus outbreak of 2009 was first reported.

Is it mere coincidence that the company also owns patents covering attenuated live viral vaccine harvesting methods along with the US government's National Institutes of Health (NIH)? Why is the US government doing business with a private military contractor accused of genocide? Or is Dyncorp colluding with the US government in a larger conspiracy?

Here is another 'coincidence'. One of the vaccine-makers awarded the contract to manufacture the much-hyped swine flu vaccine is Baxter, which is using ingredients from African green monkeys to make its vaccine in a manner explained in the Dyncorp-NIH patents!

5. Vaccines Cause The Flu

Flu shots lower natural immunity by injecting alien and toxic substances directly into the bloodstream. No other animal in the world chooses such unnatural, superficial and crude means to defend itself against invading viruses. The normal route of contact with a viral particle is via the lungs.

The vast majority of the population has a normal, healthy immune system and is perfectly capable of dealing with invaders without getting sick. But if the body's infection fighters have temporarily gone 'on strike' for reasons other than lack of a vaccine, the flu virus can gain unrestricted access to the body and cause an infection, and it should do so in order to initiate healing.

Regular vaccination (of any kind) is one of the major causes of depleted immunity. The annually administered flu shots repeatedly burden the immune system and cells of the body with foreign toxic material without giving them a chance to remove them again. The toxic viral particles can remain latent in the cells and gallstones for as long as 20 years. When they emerge, they can cause serious cell damage.

With each new vaccination, the immune system becomes more and more restricted in its effort to neutralize the live virus that suddenly appears in the blood. It may produce antibodies for the virus (although in many cases, the immune system fails to do even that), and thus subdue it. But this encounter leaves the host's immune system unnecessarily tired and weak.

It is in this context that researchers are viewing the startling results uncovered by researchers in Canada in 2009. These researchers found that people who had been vaccinated for seasonal flu were at a greater risk of catching the swine flu.

Four studies were subsequently undertaken by public health agencies in mid-2009, involving 2,700 people with and without pandemic flu or H1N1. Subjects in the first study who had taken the seasonal flu shot were observed to be at a 68 percent greater risk of contracting pandemic flu than those who had not taken the flu shot. In the other three studies, the risk was between 1.4 and 1.5 times greater. Researchers are yet to find out why this was so but they suspect that those who were at a heightened risk had weakened their immune systems by taking the seasonal flu shot prior to the swine flu outbreak.

But besides immune damage, vaccines of all kinds produce alterations in genetic material and thereby cause a whole range of malfunctions in the body, including cancerous tumors. Vaccines may even be the cause of the increasing incidence of malignant diseases in children.

Mass immunization programs have created such weak immune systems that children are even susceptible to such harmless viruses as the one causing the flu. We may have gone as far as to replace mumps and measles with cancer, leukemia, and Chronic Fatigue Syndrome.

6. Targeting The Weak

Flu vaccinations are mainly targeted at the older generation and young children. In the United Kingdom, about 10,000 people, most of them of very advanced age, (supposedly) die from flu-related illnesses. It may, therefore, sound reasonable to vaccinate the older people to protect them against the flu virus. But there is no total protection even among those who are vaccinated.

Around 20 percent or more of elderly people who get the vaccine still get a more virulent strain of flu, and many others get a lighter form of the flu. The same is true for the people in the same age group who haven't been immunized. The weak and the elderly are more likely to die from the flu, regardless of whether they have been immunized or not.

The bottom line is that there is no real advantage in taking a flu shot. And certainly, given the frailty of so many of the oldest members of society, there is absolutely no reliable way of telling whether the flu or something else may have led to their death. The death rate in and out of the flu season is actually about the same. But then, as we have seen with AIDS, statistics can be manipulated in ways that support theories which have only one objective, to keep the medical business going. For instance, when a person who is about to die anyway also catches the flu, he will be listed as a flu victim.

Instead of giving the elderly population vaccines in the misguided belief that this would take care of them, we could help them much more by improving their general resistance to disease through good diet, social engagements and exercise programs. Many elderly people do not have adequate nutrition and suffer from depression; both these factors work as powerful immune suppressants. Most of them shy away from the sun because they are being told it could cause skin cancers, especially at their age. Consequently, their vitamin D levels are among the lowest among any age group and therefore their immune system is depleted. Others don't have a warm home or they live alone.

Research has shown that these are the major risk factors for illness and death in the older generation. A series of liver cleanses alone can strengthen natural immunity, improve digestion, retard the aging process, restore health, and enhance mental functions.

In developing countries, where the elderly play an important role in society, general illness is low, provided there is enough food available. In these countries, it is more likely that old people die from malnutrition than from a strain of virus.

The elderly, of course, are one of the core target groups for the flu vaccine program. So every year we are told how older people are particularly vulnerable to the flu. We are also told that government officials are holding their breath over their fear of a devastating flu pandemic. We are even told that of the annual 36,000 flu-related deaths in the US, most of those deaths are the aged people.

The reality of the matter is quite different, though. How many people do you think died of the flu in 2009? Less than 175, according to Sherri J Tenpenny, D O, an internationally known leader in vaccine research!

Here is some more bad news for the elderly. In a damning admission in April 2010, Michael Osterholm (director, University of Minnesota's Center for Infectious Disease Research and Policy and adjunct professor in the University of Minnesota Medical School) told a conference of vaccine researchers that it was time to look for alternative solutions to safeguard senior citizens from influenza.

In his very own words: "As our immune systems deteriorate with age, the same flu vaccination that causes our bodies to mount a strong immune response in our 20s, only elicits a weak reaction in our 60s and beyond. That weaker response might be enough to offer a little protection from flu in a healthy, older person. But the evidence suggests that it's not enough to actually prevent death among most of the frail, elderly people who die each year from flu-related causes."

Now remember the swine flu hysteria, when the CDC excluded senior citizens from the first round of mass vaccination? It said this was because elderly people were at low risk of contracting the infection. Well, since then, the H1N1 swine flu antigen has been included in the trivalent seasonal flu vaccine and the CDC recommended that every citizen aged above six months be vaccinated during the 2010-2011 flu season.

Thus, not only has the CDC done a complete about-turn on the H1N1 vaccine for the elderly, it has also turned up the potency of the seasonal flu component by four times! In the CDC's words: "A higher dose formulation of an inactivated seasonal influenza vaccine for use in people age 65 years and older will be available in the 2010-2011 influenza season." The CDC also admitted that this new vaccine had not been tested and the results from trials will be available only after the 2010-2011 flu season.

And what about the other high-risk group – young children? Japanese researchers have shown that infants under one year of age fail to even generate a good antibody response following the vaccine. In the US, researchers with the International Conference of the American Thoracic Society announced their findings in May 19, 2009, which suggested that children who received the trivalent inactivated influenza vaccine (containing three strains of the flu virus) were three times more likely to be hospitalized for the flu than those who had not been vaccinated for influenza.

The researchers had followed 263 children aged between six and 18 months between 1996 and 2006. These children were regularly evaluated at the Mayo Clinic to test for laboratory-confirmed influenza.

The researchers found that not only did the flu vaccine fail to prevent the children from contracting influenza but those who did take the shot got sicker than those who did not. This has important implications for Big Pharma, which reels in big bucks while health insurance companies and parents pay for vaccines that do not work!

And here is some rather frightening news. Amid the plethora of health news being pushed onto unsuspecting parents was a news report that gave us a peek into the FDA's Dirty Tricks Department.

The July 2010 news report stated that vaccine manufacturers had begun shipping their flu vaccines for sale in the market earlier than usual due to the scare over swine flu in 2009. But it included a statement from the US FDA which stated: "The labeling for one vaccine, (Australia's) CSL Limited's Afluria, has undergone changes this season to inform health care providers about an increased incidence of fever, vomiting and febrile seizure, which was seen in young children, mainly those younger than five years, following administration of the 2010 Southern Hemisphere formulation of CSL's influenza vaccine."

As reported in WA Today: "Perth mother of two Bea Flint said her 11-month-old boy Avery had a seizure after receiving the first dose of the two-dose flu vaccination on Saturday. Mrs. Flint said that after the 9am vaccination she noticed Avery had a minor temperature about 2pm. At 7.45pm, Avery started whimpering and moaning. When Mrs. Flint got to his cot the baby had vomited and was lying on his side having a seizure. 'He couldn't cry - his head was hanging down in the car seat and he couldn't move. I was petrified - it was one of the worst experiences of my life'."

The story goes on to say, "The doctor who treated Avery told Mrs. Flint her baby was the fifth child with similar symptoms admitted to the hospital that day."

Instead of refusing to administer the potentially lethal vaccine to millions of American children, the FDA was "changing the labeling". Isn't this tantamount to culpable homicide? Mind you, the FDA also merely recommended that the vaccine maker "conduct a study on the vaccine in children". And this is the agency supposedly safeguarding our health!

All this is truly ironic, considering that the Australian government suspended all flu shots in that country after more than 250 adverse reactions, including the death of a toddler, were reported from across Australia in April 2010. These adverse events included vomiting, high fever and in some cases convulsions. Are we seeing a pattern here that vaccine-makers and the authorities refuse to admit?

211

The scare, which jammed medical hotlines, spread quickly across the country and to neighboring New Zealand as well. Australia's Health Department is on record, stating that CSL's Fluvax may be to blame even though the company denied this. CSL again!

7. The Prevention Myth

The pharmaceutical companies producing seasonal flu vaccines seem to have a more powerful effect on the population than the scientists who invented them. As early as 1980, Dr Albert Sabin, one of the world's leading virologists and a pioneer of the polio vaccine, spoke vehemently against the use of the flu vaccine, claiming that it was unnecessary for over 90 percent of the population. This, however, has not discouraged the vaccination industry to endorse vaccination for all in the name of health and protection against disease.

What makes matters worse is that there has never been a properly controlled clinical trial with the flu vaccine. Because we don't know anything about its long-term effects, we may be unknowingly producing generations of people with debilitated immune systems and chronic diseases.

Flu vaccination is an unproved and unscientific practice and nothing in the scientific literature can certify or guarantee its safety. Whereas it is illegal to put mercury or formaldehyde into food products because these are proven to have lethal effects, it is perfectly legal to inject the same toxins into the blood of millions of people, year after year. Just because it is legal to poison the population one shot a time, it doesn't make it safe. The most safe and effective way to fight infections, including the flu, is to prevent it. There is no substitute for a health-increasing regimen.

Vaccination, on the other hand, offers no real protection. Injecting the body with foreign and poisonous viral material is counterproductive to improving our well-being. Dr John Seal from the American National Institute for Allergies and Infectious Diseases warns that we have to assume that every flu vaccination can cause the Guillain-Barré Syndrome. In this sense, prevention is not better than cure.

To those who recently heard the mass media report about a British study that claims flu vaccines can reduce the risk of heart attacks by as much as 19 percent, I have to say that this was a clever marketing ploy and is pure misinformation. What the media reported is not what the researchers told them. The study looked at the records of 79,000 patients age 40 or older in England and Wales from 2001 to 2007 and allegedly found that those who had received flu shots had fewer heart attacks. No true link was established, though, because, as it turned out, there is none. USA Today reported that there were noticeable flaws in the study.

"Dr. Kirk Garratt, associate director of the division of cardiac intervention at Lenox Hill Hospital in New York City, said the study found there were 19 percent fewer heart attack patients vaccinated in the previous year, not that there was a 19 percent reduction in heart attacks among the vaccinated," USA Today said.

"If getting a flu shot could prevent 19 percent of heart attacks, it would have been noticed before now," Garratt added.

Who doesn't want to reduce his risk of having a heart attack? There are millions of concerned people out there who want to feel safe, and if their safety depends on receiving a flu shot, they will have one. It is a sad fact that so many people blindly follow the advice contained in such powerful and persuasive media headlines, "Flu Shots lower your risk of heart attack".

As Dr. Kirk Garratt told the USA Today: "This study did not measure risk of heart attack in vaccinated and non-vaccinated people. It measured rates of vaccination among heart attack patients and those without heart attack."

Of course, the study found that 19 percent fewer heart attack patients received flu shots in the previous year – which does not equate with the 19 percent reduction in heart attacks among those vaccinated, as the media headlines wanted us to believe.

The bottom line is that flu shots have neither been shown to lessen one's chances of becoming infected with a flu virus, nor reduce inflammation of arteries or the number of related pneumonia cases, or pneumonia-linked deaths (which the CDC tends to refer to as "flu deaths").

A 2008 study published in the Lancet, and confirming an earlier study published in May 2003 in the New England Journal of Medicine, found that vaccinating against influenza failed to reduce the risk of pneumonia in elderly people. The latter study also found that no association existed between pneumococcal vaccination and a reduced risk of pneumonia from any cause.

Since inflammation is a key factor involved in increasing heart attack risk, and vaccines actually increase inflammation in the body, I therefore caution everyone with a heart condition, cancer, arthritis or other to stay away from flu vaccines or any other vaccine.

Chapter 9

The Whole Truth

Have you ever said you've had a "gut feeling"? Or that you feel a "soulful connection" with something? If you have, then there, in that very moment, you experienced the mind-body connection at work.

But in quite the opposite way, modern medicine, and most people as well, look at the human body as a collection of parts. According to this mechanistic view, when 'one part' of the body malfunctions, it needs to be fixed. Enter the doctor's world and you will see his arsenal of sophisticated tools – drugs, gizmos, surgery, and even new body parts! Or check out the army of specialists – cardiologists, gastroenterologists, oncologists, diabetologists, neurologists, dermatologists, and the like.

Over the years, technology has made giant strides, and medical science began to rely – nay, pride itself – more and more on high-tech diagnostic and treatment tools. So today, it is not enough for a doctor to specialize in one organ or system of the body. Thus enter the tribe of 'super-specialists', who focus on micro-aspects of body parts, organs and processes. Thus, we have impressive sounding super-specialties which sound something like this: cardiac anaesthesia, vitreo-retinal surgery, interventional cardiology and hemato-oncology. The greater the degree of 'specialization', the more 'prestigious' the doctor. Thus goes the pecking order in modern medicine.

Apart from the confusing – and dubious – nature of these terms, super-speciality medicine is the antithesis of mind-body or holistic medicine. The former views disease as a flaw in a body part or a bio-physiological system. Hence, much like a car that has broken down, the solution to illness and disease is to treat or remove the malfunctioning body part and replace it with a new one. At least, that's what the 'super-specialists' believe.

But why only medicine? Modern society too is going the super-specialty way. Tasks at work have become so complex that they need to be broken down into simpler units. Thus we need specialists or super-specialists for each aspect of each task, whether it is the world of finance, information technology, fashion, film-making and even cooking!

Take the way we live, for example. The human body is made up of around 70 percent water and we, like all other species, are creatures of the earth. But modern urban lifestyles, which most of us treasure and even exalt, have taken us so far from nature that many of us forget where we came from and our umbilical connection with the planet.

We tend to live in a cocooned world, overstimulating ourselves with work, entertainment and other forms of stress, and still expect to be healthy and happy. Even 'time' is dissected and fragmented to an extreme. Which is why we have 'work time', 'family time', 'quality time', 'free time', 'no time', and so many other types of 'time'. It boggles the mind!

The starting point to living healthy and happily begins with the question: are you in tune with your inner self, your surroundings and the universe at large? The answer to health or to ill-health on the flipside, lies in the answer to that singular question.

Think about it. Does your brain or liver work in isolation? Is there really a separation between the large intestine, small intestine and gall bladder? Just as your body parts function in exquisite union, your physiological and thought processes too are intimately connected to each other. On another level, your mind and body mesh in subtle and not-so-subtle ways with your environment, the people around you and your daily activities. You mind and body are also connected to and constantly reacting to events that occurred way back in the past, some you may no longer remember.

There are many layers and levels on which we function at all times, whether we are aware of them or not. Illness, disease and immunity work in the very same way. Did you know that your immune system is finely tuned to your stress levels? Why else do you think 'worry warts' are more prone to falling ill? Why else do people with no personal or family history of heart disease and no sign of arterial obstruction suddenly collapse from a heart attack?

Scientists are now talking about cellular memory. Still in the realm of 'theory', this is an area of research that assumes that it is not just the brain but our organs too that store memories, habits, tastes and interests. They believe that neuropeptides – small specialized protein molecules – which help the brain signal and communicate with various organs are involved in cellular memory.

This was assumed with the discovery that neuropeptides, once thought to be present in the brain, are also present in some organs of the human body, especially the heart. Before you leap to any conclusions, allow me to clarify that I am not offering this as 'evidence' of a mind-body connection. I am merely suggesting that there is much more to the functioning of the human body, even individual body parts, than even modern science can explain.

Hence, not only is the reductionist view of modern medicine the polar opposite of holistic medicine, I believe it is not even necessary to 'prove' the mind-body link. All we need to know that it is there, it exists and that it influences us in everything we do, whether we realize it or not.

1. Mind Over Matter

Disease is a product of fragmentation of the self, something that takes place when the body is not working like the fine-tuned machine that it is designed to be. It takes place when we are far from our optimal level of functioning, which invariably causes an organ or system to malfunction.

This is because in order to stay healthy, the body *needs* to maintain its unity and harmony. Let us look at this in another way by focusing on 'balance'. Every ecosystem, all ecosystems together, life and the universe itself all require a certain equilibrium or balance of energy to function optimally.

Therefore, when the body and mind are in a state of balance and unity, you are in a state of good health. You also experience a sense of inner peace or serenity. Most people do not experience a sense of perfect harmony and unity but their mind, body and energy work in a fairly unified way. We label people like this as 'balanced', 'practical' and 'grounded' and we like being around them simply because they exude a sense of easy calm. The odds are they are also in a state of good health and maintain a sense of mental and physical balance despite the rigors of modern living and the umpteen tasks they need to perform.

On the other hand, there are those who live in a perpetual state of chaos and their energy is in constant turmoil. We call people like this 'chaotic' or 'extremists'. But chaos may also manifest itself in subtle ways. It doesn't necessarily show up as a chaotic mind or people who we label as 'disorganized'. Remember, the criterion for chaos used here is a mind that is in conflict and in a state of fragmentation. The body then uses all the energy it can muster from various sources to maintain the unity and integrity of the mind.

When it is unable to keep it all together, something gives way. This is when disease manifests itself, first as symptoms such as sleep loss, weight loss or abnormal weight gain, falling hair, clammy and sweaty hands, skin eruptions, and shallow breathing. It is a state where the body uses up and depletes the body's physical reserves, which are meant to be drawn upon every now and then to resolve conflicts and meet stressful situations. The constant depletion of energy alters normal metabolic and physiological processes.

Tremendous amounts of mental energy are used up in the process, which is why some people become seemingly obsessed with certain issues while others become listless and depressed. Note, the very same process takes place on a subconscious level too. It is here that past conflicts continue to exist and take a toll without a conscious trace!

On a more everyday level, have you noticed that when you are stressed, you lose your appetite, you are restless and you are unable to sleep well? You are also preoccupied with whatever it is that is stressing you out, perhaps a challenging task at work, a tough life choice, conflicts with your children or financial worries.

When the conflict or crisis is either resolved or it passes, you literally begin to 'breathe easy'. That's more than just a metaphor. Your breathing processes normalize, blood circulation improves and you feel more energized. This happens because the extra energy the mind and body harnessed to focus on the problem is released back into the bodily processes that they were drawn from and the balance is restored.

It is in this context that I find Dr Ryke Geerd Hamer's Germanic/German New Medicine (GNM) revolutionary. According to Dr Hamer, microbes and other pathogens do not cause disease; psychological conflicts do. Germs, on the other hand, have a role to play only in the healing phase of an illness.

As incredible as this may sound, Dr Hamer's research is scientifically documented and provides further proof of the mind-body connection and the powerful role our perceptions and conflicts play in the development of disease including cancer.

According to Dr Hamer, whose system of medicine is explained by Five Biological Laws, every conflict or 'conflict-shock' leads to the formation of concentric circles or rings in specific areas of the brain, causing a 'lesion' visible on a CT scan. At the time of the shock, the collection of brain cells in the area that is affected relays the shock to the specific organ whose functions it controls. According to Dr Hamer, this is the genesis of disease.

He points out that the human being is a product of evolution and hence he says the brain interprets conflict and shock in evolutionary ways as all animals are genetically programmed to react to these stimuli in set and predictable ways for survival purposes.

Hence, according to Dr Hamer, all types of conflicts may be classified into a few categories only, in evolutionary terms. And these categories are linked to specific brain areas. Dr Hamer divides the brain into two parts – the 'old brain' (brain stem and cerebellum), which is concerned with basic survival issues that relate to breathing, eating or reproduction; and the 'new brain' (cerebrum), which is concerned with more advanced issues such as territorial conflict, separation conflict, identity conflict and self-devaluation conflict.

Since each type of conflict relates to specific areas of the brain and each area of the brain is linked to a specific set of organs and systems, the nature of the psychological conflict or shock impacts on a specific organ in the body. According to Dr Hamer, if the old brain is involved, the organs and tissues affected are those controlled by the old brain including the lungs, liver, colon, prostate, uterus, corium skin, pleura, peritoneum, pericardium, breast glands, etc.

On the other hand, organs and tissues controlled by the new brain include the ovaries, testicles, bones, lymph nodes, epidermis, the lining of the cervix, bronchial tubes, coronary vessels, milk ducts, etc.

Again, whether the organ responds with cell proliferation (tumors) or tissue meltdown (ulcers, lesions, etc) or organ malfunction depends on whether old or new brain areas are affected, and this, in turn, depends on the nature of the conflict.

Hence, according to Dr Hamer, conflict is both psychological and biological and it is at the confluence of these two levels that disease originates. Flip that around and one can say that disease is caused by conflict, which impacts on the physical and biological level and must be understood in the evolutionary context.

Animals are devoid of 'higher' intellectual functions and their psychological conflict and biological shock invariably relates to territorial loss, loss of the nest or an offspring, separation from their mate or the herd, sudden starvation or a fight-flight situation.

All our psychological traumas, anxieties, depression and diseases can be classified into these seemingly simple categories. For instance, loss of a mortgaged home or infidelity relate to territory and separation from one's mate as in betrayal or the death of a loved one.

Of course, what is traumatic for one individual need not be traumatic for another. Hence, conflict is highly subjective and depends on temperament, upbringing, coping mechanisms, perceptions, attitudes and values, morals, one's state of physical health and genetic predisposition. But, according to Dr Hamer, once a perceived conflict or shock does occur, it impacts in a definite and predetermined way on the body.

According to GNM, healing or recovery is the second stage of disease, where the tissue, organ or system that is affected reverses the processes produced by the initial shock. Hence, in the case of cancer, which involves a proliferation of cells (a protective mechanism to help the affected organ cope), healing is characterized by infection and subsequent tissue meltdown.

On the other hand, in the case of ulcers or tissue damage, the affected area is refilled with cells and tissue, which may initially result in swelling, spasms, itching and inflammation. That is why you sometimes have to 'get worse' before you get better.

As mentioned earlier, microbes such as bacteria and viruses, which are invariably blamed as the cause of disease, kick in to heal an affected organ or body part after the conflict that caused it is resolved.

According to Dr Hamer, pathogens such as fungi and bacteria help in healing only old brain disorders while viruses are play a part in healing new brain diseases. These microbes decompose tumors and damaged tissue that are now not needed by the body. That is why vaccination, chemotherapy and antibiotics are harmful – they thwart healing.

Hence, diseases such as the flu, hepatitis, herpes and stomach flu, which are typically accompanied by swelling, fever, pus, discharge, pain and the like are a sign that a 'virulent' but natural healing process is running its course.

Dr Hamer points out that since conventional medicine witnesses the action of microbes and their effects on the body only during the 'virulent' phase (which is actually the healing process), it blames these pathogens for causing disease.

Recent research has produced stunning evidence suggesting that individuals who have cancer but live in a socially enriched environment may be able to heal themselves. Spontaneous regression is not a new phenomenon and has been observed in certain types of cancers such as neuroblastoma, renal cell carcinoma, lymphoma, malignant melanoma and certain types of breast cancer.

Now, researchers from Ohio State University may have found out just why and how spontaneous regression takes place. According to findings published in the journal *Cell*, studies on mice found that cancerous tumors in rodents shrank considerably when these rodents were placed in an environment with more toys and more mice to interact with. Tumors in these 'enriched' mice were found to have shrunk 77 percent in mass and 43 percent in volume compared to mice in the control group.

Attempting to find out what changes had taken place at the biochemical level, researchers found that the 'enriched' mice had higher levels of glucosteroids in their blood. This suggested that they had experienced greater stress than their control counterparts but the nature of their stress seems to have mattered – 'happy stress'!

In addition to this, the 'enriched' mice exhibited certain metabolic changes and also displayed higher levels of a growth factor released from the hypothalamus called brain-derived neurotrophic factor (BDNF). Further investigation showed that an increase in BDNF levels correlated with a reduction in the tumors.

In recent times, there has been a lot of debate on whether screening for cancer – especially mammograms in women – is a good idea at all. The debate centers on the fact that some types of cancers – kidney, testicular, lymphoma and melanoma – often undergo spontaneous regression. While this is a fact that many oncologists will confirm, some estimate that as many as 1 in every 400 such cases disappear on their own. In fact, around 20 percent of 'low-grade, B-cell, Non-Hodgkin's lymphoma cases disappear on their own and oncologists prefer not to treat these cancers unless they turn aggressive.

Conventional medicine is yet to find the key to unlocking the 'mystery' of spontaneous regression. But the answer is no mystery at all. While cancer and the mind are both extremely complex phenomena and highly subjective, the fact is that self-healing is not only possible but it does take place in serious diseases such as cancer as well. In my book, *Cancer is not a Disease*, I go even further and actually claim that cancer is a healing or survival mechanism that needs to be supported, not intercepted by harsh and destructive medical treatments.

Also, the study by the Ohio State University researchers throws light on another powerful factor that influences not only our health but serious illnesses such as cancer – social factors and the 'happiness quotient'.

Autoimmune disorders, immunodeficiency and immune disorders are another class of disease that is on the rise. In these diseases, the immune system of the individual malfunctions and, according to conventional medicine, the body begins to attack itself.

Let us return to GNM and how it views autoimmune diseases. Historically, these disorders made their appearance relatively recently. They became increasingly common during the 20th century, during the Industrial Revolution, not because of the unhealthy conditions that people were forced to live and work in but due to the sudden and phenomenal increase of the middle and wealthy classes.

Immune disorders are indeed an affliction of the wealthy and educated, people who as a group tend to have more to fear than others. I am not suggesting that fears and worries are the curse of the economically endowed, just that the greater the education level, the greater the probability that they have sedentary lives and jobs.

This, in evolutionary language, means that people who don't go out there and 'get their hands dirty' have less than capable coping mechanisms. And this, in turn, means that they have more to worry about and fear from their environment.

People who live with fear and mistrust of the environment attempt to control their surroundings instead of getting to the root of their problems and solving them. Hence, every sign and symptom of disease is met with increasing fear – a sort of reaction to their own reactions. Eventually, the origin of the disease is so far removed from the self that conflict resolution is seemingly impossible, at least not without intervention.

The vicious cycle is: Disease causes fear, which causes more disease and eventually leads to a breakdown of the immune system, which is so weakened that it cannot cope. There simply isn't enough coping power. In other words, the greater the worry and anxiety, the greater the conflict-shock, the less able is the body to cope, and thus the vicious cycle continues.

Therefore, according to New German Medicine, autoimmune diseases such as AIDS are a combination of symptoms resulting from multiple conflict-shocks.

2. You Are Your Own Doctor

New German Medicine and other similar ways of looking at disease have completely transformed the way we define health. Unfortunately, we have distanced ourselves so much from our true nature and 'modern medicine' has seduced us so much through propaganda and advertisements that we measure health in terms of tests, scans and biopsies.

You don't need to assess your health by a series of blood pressure readings, the amount of LDL or HDL cholesterol in your blood or your blood sugar levels. The healthiest way to assess your health and well-being is to assess your quality of life. This means respecting your body, treating it right, breathing easy, sleeping and eating well, spending time in the sun and nature, playing with children, and enjoying the feeling of energy and vitality and energy when your body and mind are 'happy'. (For more on how to rejuvenate yourself with healthy lifestyle choices, you may wish to read *Timeless Secrets of Rejuvenation and Health*)

Keeping good health also means enjoying a walk in the park, having a good time with family and friends, playing with a pet, achieving your goals and being happy at work and everything else you do. Good health therefore means maintaining a sense of balance in your life in all aspects – in your habits, choices, attitudes, wants and desires, etc while making that life-changing connection between the mind and body.

I can tell you this: When you achieve all or even most of the above, you will intuitively *know* you are on the right track. What if I were to tell you that you are your best healer? That your doctor is actually inside you? That the best and most lasting healing comes from within? Learning to trust your intuitive wisdom beats any blood pressure or treadmill test.

What this boils down to is the positive or negative energy you experience and radiate. It is this energy – which translates into very definite positive or negative chemical reactions in your body – which can either heal you and keep you healthy or make you ill. Falling ill then serves you with the opportunity to return to a state of balance and harmony.

When was the last time you felt grateful for what you have? A lot of people are simply too preoccupied with what they *don't* have. It is easy to feel self-pity or an overarching sense of ambition or to 'achieve' in order to compensate for what one doesn't have. How about what you *do* have? However, when you re-focus your thoughts on the positive – and gratitude is a great place to start – you basically realign your energy. And *that's* good health.

Health means wholeness. By accepting what is with gratitude, regardless of whether it is positive or negative, you become whole again, and healing can take place naturally. On the other hand, fighting or resisting anything, whether it is another person or a disease, leaves you subjected to fear and fragmented. It is a difficult position to be in if you want the body to heal and become whole again. Being diagnosed with cancer can cause you to fall apart, lose your sleep, appetite, weight, and your joy of life. It can leave you with such an intense fear of death that it can literally eat you up alive (called wasting) and kill you. Cancer doesn't do this, but the diagnosis of cancer can easily do that. Getting the certainly that you have cancer is soon replaced with the uncertainly of what it will do to you. Once again, it is difficult to heal while feeling threatened.

Alas, most of us, brainwashed by doctors, their gadgetry and apparent wizardry, have placed the center of control outside ourselves and into the hands of physicians and the pharmaceutical industry. Handing over our power to pills, vaccines, or men in white coats will rob us of the power that our body requires to heal itself. But pause for a while and ponder the many miracles that are taking place inside your body, whether you're conscious of them or not.

For instance, when you sleep, millions of cells in your body are being repaired; toxins are being carried away from tissues through your lymph and blood to your liver to be processed and prepared for excretion; the food you ate for lunch and dinner is undergoing the amazingly complex process of digestion; and new skin is growing on an elbow you grazed against a bookshelf – all of this without you even consciously experiencing it.

The body basically carries out the processes of healing whether you are aware of them or not. That's because **the body has a basic, innate and automatic tendency to heal itself, to be whole and to be unified (versus being fragmented)**. As I have explained earlier (See Chapter 1: *The Vaccine Myth*), even disease is a process of healing. Acknowledging this, becoming aware of these processes and being grateful for them is part of becoming and staying healthy.

Instead, we assault our body in so many ways which thwart good health and healing – overdependence on processed foods, over-stimulating ourselves (who said multi-tasking was a virtue?) in so many ways, and becoming pill poppers at the drop of the hat. Yet, our bodies soldier on, taking the stress of the daily assault in stoic silence. How ungrateful we are!

If you listen to your body, it will tell you what it needs. What we often call disease – high blood pressure, asthma, diabetes, obesity and allergies – are actually signals that the body is off-balance and needs rebalancing through diet, rehydration, sunshine or a change in sleep pattern.

But when ill, most people reach for a bottle of pills and other chemical formulations. These drugs, painkillers and surgery have just the opposite effect. They shut down your symptoms (which are actually signs that the body is undergoing healing), or leave you incomplete when you cut out a body part. Most approaches of modern medicine take you only deeper into a diseased state and switch off the power to self-heal. Not surprising, since published research shows that 90 percent of these approaches don't work and are not backed by scientific evidence. On the other hand, there are many natural ways to cleanse and rebalance your body and reverse seemingly incurable conditions such cancer and autoimmune diseases.

Therefore, at the center of this self-healing is the belief that your body can return to a state of optimal functioning and will not let you down. All you need to do is switch on. Supporting evidence for self-healing comes from another tool routinely used by scientific researchers. Only, they seem to be missing the point! It is called the 'placebo effect'. As discussed before, a placebo is a 'sugar pill' given to a group of subjects in an experiment while another group – the experimental group – is administered the 'real' medicine which is being tested. The assumption is that since both groups are given a pill, both groups have been treated equally and hence any difference that may arise in the experimental group will be due to the 'real drug' that was administered.

But the 'placebo effect' is a phenomenon where individuals who are given nothing more than a sugar pill show evidence of healing simply because they believe they are under treatment and that the treatment will cure them.

Now be careful you don't miss the point – which is the belief of the patient that the drug (or placebo), an operation or a treatment program will relieve pain or cure illness. Deep trust or a sure feeling of recovery is all that one has at one's disposal to initiate a healing response. Drawing upon the powerful mind-body connection, one releases natural opioids (morphine-type painkillers) from areas of the brain that are activated by certain thought processes. The corresponding neurotransmitters for pain relief are known as endorphins. Endorphins are about 40,000 times more powerful than even heroin or morphine.

A patient who develops a cancerous growth may start producing extra amounts of Interleukin II and Interferon to destroy the tumor cells. Being products of DNA, the body can make these anti-cancer drugs in every cell and eradicate cancer in a moment (spontaneous regression), provided one knows how to trigger their release. The triggers are trust, confidence and happiness, the very same triggers that cause the placebo effect.

Your body is capable of manufacturing every drug that could possibly be produced by the pharmaceutical industry. Synthetically derived drugs only 'work' because the cells of your body have receptors for some of the chemicals contained in these drugs. This means that the body is capable of making these chemicals too. Otherwise, these receptors wouldn't exist.

The body knows how to make them with the utmost precision, in the correct dosage and with perfect timing. The body's own drugs cost us nothing and they have no harmful side effects. Pharmaceutical drugs, on the other hand, are very expensive and much less specific or accurate. In addition, the side effects they produce usually end up being more severe than the ailments for which they are used.

What makes matters worse is that an estimated 35-45 percent of all prescriptions have no specific effect on the disease for which they are prescribed. The bottom line is that the positive results are largely and directly caused by the body's own healing response or are triggered by the placebo effect. They have nothing to do with the medical treatment itself.

The placebo effect is often experienced in another situation. Doctors too have the power to inspire in their patients the confidence to believe that they are receiving the most suitable and best treatment available for their ailments. The expectation of finding relief may be the main motivation behind a patient visiting the doctor. Also, the doctor is likely to believe that his prescription will produce the desired effect, that is, relieve his patient's symptoms.

The combined belief of the doctor in his treatment and the trust and faith the patient places in the doctor can produce a 'medicine' that is capable of transforming even a useless treatment or a non-specific drug into a dynamo of healing. This can very well lead to a definite *improvement of the treated condition, and in some cases, a complete cure. Here, 'medicine' is nothing but the placebo effect.*

If the doctor is convinced that the treatment of the patient's illness will be successful, the patient's perception of the doctor's confidence is much more likely to produce a placebo response than if the doctor is doubtful about his approach. In other words, if a doctor can inspire a patient to believe that he is going to improve, he has done a much better job than any sophisticated treatment may be able to accomplish.

That is why a warm-hearted, honest and optimistic doctor who listens to his intuition and feels both compassion and love for his fellow human beings is not only preferred by patients but is most likely to be an effective healer, regardless of the medication he prescribes for the ailment. We usually call this 'bedside manner'.

The current tendency of an increasing number of people to seek alternative practitioners is not so much based on what they offer to a patient. Rather, it is a matter of how they make their patients feel. The fact that alternative therapists use mostly natural methods and compounds for their treatments makes natural therapies more acceptable to the patient than medical treatments. It also makes their approaches more humane and potentially more powerful as placebos.

We all have a preprogrammed natural instinct to know what is good and useful for us, although many people have managed to subdue it. This is possibly one reason why natural cures work so well. It is a gut-level healing effect produced when we eat pure, fresh foods, healing herbs and other natural remedies. A herb from the Himalayan mountains or a piece of ginger is more likely to trigger a placebo response in us than the synthetic fat Olestra or a pharmaceutical drug used to reduce blood pressure. Natural things are naturally pleasing to the body and mind. It is no wonder that a naturopath has become a symbol of natural healing.

The key to healing is therefore faith, trust and a belief that one will get well, and that if disease strikes, this constitutes the body's best and most efficient way of restoring balance, health and vitality.

3. Placebo Fraud Invalidates Most Clinical Trials

Apparently, nobody saw this coming, except in 1998, in the first edition of my book Timeless Secrets of Health and Rejuvenation, I wrote extensively about the underlying fraud committed during pharmaceutical studies that involve a placebo group. However, the following new findings published by researchers at the University of

California in the October 2010 issue of the Annals of Internal Medicine, takes the scientific fraud committed by drug companies to an entirely new level.

The research which was funded by the University of California Foundation Fund 3929 – Medical Reasoning, basically revealed that almost all clinical trials comparing pharmaceutical drugs to placebo pills are unscientifically invalid because the placebos used in these studies weren't valid placebos at all. The study entitled "What's in Placebos: Who Knows? Analysis of Randomized, Controlled Trials" was led by Beatrice A. Golomb, MD, PhD. Because the placebos used in the studies weren't really placebos at all, this rendered the studies scientifically invalid.

The background argument of the University of California study states: "No regulations govern placebo composition. The composition of placebos can influence trial outcomes and merits reporting."

In the study, the researchers reviewed 167 placebo-controlled trials published in peer-reviewed medical journals in 2008 and 2009 and found that the lead researchers of 92 percent of those trials never even disclosed the ingredients of their placebo pills.

Why is this so relevant? Because the only way to determine drug efficacy is to compare it to an inactive, inert substance (placebo). Since there are no FDA regulations governing placebo composition (I wonder why), according to the study's background statement, "the composition of placebos can influence trial outcomes and merits reporting". In other words, the kind of placebo used during a clinical trial can pretty much determine the 'effectiveness' of the pharmaceutical drug in question.

In truth, there are no inert placebos. Every substance, pill powder or liquid, has some specific effect on the body. Simple sugar, for example, raises blood sugar levels almost immediately. So, in a clinical trial done on diabetics, the placebo group that receives an inert sugar pill will, of course, fare much worse than the group that receives the actual medication consisting of hypoglycemic agents which are claimed to lower blood sugar levels. It doesn't take much to proof that the drug is an effective one to help diabetics control their blood sugar.

Likewise, there are placebos used in heart studies. These 'inert' placebo capsules may consist of partially-hydrogenated oils containing trans fatty acids which are known to seriously injure coronary arteries and the heart. Naturally, a totally useless heart drug will come out as the winner, defeating the placebo by leaps and bounds.

According to the University of California study, only 8 percent of clinical trials disclosed the list the placebo ingredients. The lacking FDA rules allow pharmaceutical companies to scheme up the perfect placebo responsible to make the placebo look ridiculously ineffective when compared with the medical drug. The FDA requires a drug to work just 5 percent better than a placebo to give it the approval stamp. This is easily achieved by choosing a placebo that makes the studied drug look good.

Most drug trials are funded by drug giants and conducted by scientists sponsored by them. By not regulating the placebos, the FDA provides the drug companies with a legitimate loophole to conduct drug trials with a pre-determined outcome. The only potential obstacle they can face is when the tested drug is so extremely toxic that it seriously harms a large number of subjects, more than in the placebo group. This has been shown in a number of diabetes and arthritis trials where too many subjects died as a result of ingesting the real drugs.

The bottom line is that the placebos are typically provided by the same companies that fund the clinical trials, meaning, by those who will benefit mostly from a successful outcome. It is at the discretion of the drug makers to determine what kind of placebo pills they need in order to fake their clinical trials and turn their initial investments into massive income streams.

Ironically, this completely unscientific, misleading and criminal practice is considered to be "the gold standard of scientific evidence".

Medicals scientists who denounce and ridicule the methods of alternative or integrative medicine, such as homeopathy, Ayurveda, Chinese medicine, acupuncture, etc often claim the above method of scientific investigation (that uses a result-friendly placebo) to be the only valid research method there is, while being the worst offenders of objective scientific investigation. As it turns out, the greatest quackery ever committed is by the scientists behind these trials, and the doctors and health agencies that use these results to justify their useless (unproven) and potentially harmful medical treatments. Medical science has become the biggest fraud mankind has ever witnessed.

The often cited "scientific evidence" is based on scientific manipulation or placebo fraud. If a placebo used during a trial isn't a real placebo at all but a substance that can alter the results in favor of a studied drug, then the "scientific evidence" is a just a fraud. When you go to your doctor and he gives you a prescription medication claiming that studies have proven it to be effective for your particular disorder, he intentionally or unwittingly commits fraud. He is practically selling you a snake oil that was produced by a corrupt drug maker and labeled as medicine. As the New England Journal of Medicine and the WHO once admitted, 85-90 percent of what is being offered at hospitals or doctors' offices today is not backed by scientific evidence.

Just stating that a particular substance - such as sugar, oil, a synthetic chemical, fluoridated water, calcium carbonate (chalk dust), or any one of dozens of different metallic minerals and chemicals - is inert and can be used as a placebo is not enough to make it inert. It is wishful thinking. But wishful thinking is exactly what the trial researchers do when they compare a drug with such a 'scientific' placebo. Not only do they receive full approval of such misuse of the placebo by their colleagues, the Federal Drug Administration, but as a reward, their 'work' is also published in prestigious medical journals.

Dr Beatric Golomb said, "We can only hope that this hasn't seriously systematically affected medical treatment." Millions of people take prescription drugs every day that have never been proven to be more effective than hope or faith, which is the power behind a placebo pill. However, these drugs can have devastating and potentially lethal side effects, while faith and hope do no harm. Over 100,000 people die each year in the US alone from drug related side effects.

Drug makers are often very unscrupulous, and it is irrelevant to them how many people die at their hands. They are only held responsible by their shareholders, and as long as they make a lot of money, it is all that counts. If they choose a placebo that is harming subjects, the trial will bring about the project better and faster 'positive' results.

For example, during trials testing new AIDS drugs, researchers use lactose as the preferred placebo. They know very well that most AIDS patients are lactose intolerant. This placebo can seriously affect their immune system, which is already highly compromised in AIDS patients. It's like conducting a clinical trial on a drug that suppresses brain hormones associated with alcohol addiction, during which the researchers hand out placebo pills that contain alcohol. The FDA hasn't made any effort to rule against this unethical practice.

Sometimes, clinical trial researchers get caught in their ruthless unethical schemes, such as the well-known Dr Scott Ruben who was believed to be one of the best researchers among his peers. Although he faked at least 21 clinical trials and published the fake results in the most prestigious medical journals, doctors still write millions of prescriptions for these unproven drugs, or rather, snake oils. It doesn't matter that the drugs don't help anyone as long as it is good for the economy. Drug giants are just too big to fail. Imagine if the junk science that backs the pharmaceutical industry were to be outlawed, there would hardly be a medical drug on the market, and much of the medical industry would collapse.

4. A Little Sunshine, Please!

One way to flip the healing switch is to make sure you get enough sunlight. Sunlight is one of those things that we overlook or take for granted perhaps *because* it is free, yet it is a life-giving force that sustains all life on the planet. Nature does not make mistakes and there must be a very good reason why the human species is meant to live under the protective umbrella of the sun.

Let me flip the argument. Why is it that people who live indoors a lot are more prone to falling ill? Why does the flu strike people who live in temperate regions more than in the tropics? The common thread here is sunlight. Urban lifestyles have become so indoors-oriented that we seem to duck the sun at every opportunity.

We leave home for work in our cars (with sunscreen shades or glass that blocks out UV rays), spend an entire work day in a temperature-controlled environment, drive back home or catch the tube under similar circumstances and then sink down in front of a television screen or computer monitor in our homes in the evening. For those who do spend a fair amount of time outdoors, wearing shades is chic and whether faced with blinding glare or not, it is a must. The point I am making is simply this: we simply do not expose out bodies to enough sunlight.

But why is sunlight so important? In the context of health and immunity, sunlight catalyses the synthesis of Vitamin D, which plays a role in various processes in the human body including the synthesis of enzymes, hormones and neurotransmitters. It is crucial for calcium absorption and strengthening the body's immune response.

Did you know that Vitamin D plays a crucial role in preventing cancer, osteoporosis and depression and helps keep modern scourges such as diabetes and obesity at bay? It prevents infectious diseases far more effectively than vaccines could ever hope to. But before we discuss that, let's first look at various aspects of Vitamin D.

Vitamin D is present in some foods but you cannot get the quantities your body requires from your diet. The best and most reliable way to get enough Vitamin D is to expose yourself to a moderate amount of sunlight daily. Sunlight 'throws the switch' that kicks off the synthesis of the vitamin in your skin.

It is the ultraviolet band in sunlight that activates Vitamin D and sets off a complex chain reaction involving your kidneys and liver, which convert inactive Vitamin D into its active form – an active hormone called calcitriol.

Among its major benefits, Vitamin D helps the body maintain the balance of calcium and phosphorus that it requires. It also helps the body absorb calcium. This why Vitamin D is critical to healthy bones and teeth. Individuals who are Vitamin D-deprived have brittle bones. Such children may suffer from rickets (which is now making a huge comeback), while adults may suffer from osteoporosis. Deficiencies may also result in asthma, allergies, Alzheimer's disease, gluten intolerance, learning and behavior disorders, autoimmune disorders and Parkinson's Disease. (For more on the benefits of sunlight and Vitamin D, you can read my book, *Heal Yourself With Sunlight*)

How Much Vitamin D?: Just 20 minutes in the noon sun, three to four times a week is all the ultraviolet light your body needs. That there is no substitute for this is evident from the fact that you cannot get the required amounts of Vitamin D from foods. Some foods that contain Vitamin D are fatty fish such as salmon, cod and mackerel. Not only are these fish not eaten often but you would need to eat them several times a week to get an adequate amount of Vitamin D.

Others believe fortified milk and orange juice will suffice. But the truth is that you would need to drink ten glasses of milk or orange juice daily for your body to get as much of the vitamin as it needs. Multivitamins too are not half as useful as sunlight as they give you less than half your requirement while promoting the quick-fix myth of good health.

Just as sunlight exposure varies from one individual to another, people living on different continents are exposed to different amounts and patterns of sunlight. Simply put: The farther you live from the equator, the less sunlight (UV rays) you are exposed to and the more likely you are to suffer from a Vitamin D deficiency. However, those living at high elevations such as the mountains of Switzerland enjoy higher concentrations of UV light and tend to have healthier vitamin D levels.

It gets worse in winter, when sunlight is very weak. The best way around this problem is to get enough sunlight in the summer and spring months, and use a vitamin D lamp or UV lamp during the colder months. Taking a vacation in a warm, sunny, country during the winter also helps. When your body synthesizes enough Vitamin D, it stores the excess in your fat and releases it when levels dip. This presents a problem for individuals who are obese, where the adipose doesn't seem to be able to release the stored Vitamin D.

Also, if your body has made enough of the vitamin during the summer, stores will last for around three months before turning deficient. You could also take a Vitamin D supplement during those cold and dark winter months, but this can be risky. You will need to carefully monitor your blood levels to make sure you do not overdose on Vitamin D which, if ingested orally, can act as a poison and even kill you. If this vitamin is produced in response to sunlight, the body monitors its levels and makes sure you never have too much of it in the blood.

Skin color also affects Vitamin D production in your body. Darker skins need about 20 to 30 times more sunlight exposure than people who are pale and very light-skinned. Make sure you don't get sunburned, though. As soon as your skin starts reddening, it is an indication that you have filled your requirement for vitamin D. But also make sure you do not use sunscreen and sunglasses or it will defeat the very purpose! As explained in my book *Heal Yourself with Sunlight*, sunglasses interfere with the secretion of an important brain hormone that regulates melanin production in the skin, which, in turn, is needed to protect your skin against damage from the Ultraviolet A radiation.

The shocking truth is that around 40 percent of Americans suffer from a deficiency in Vitamin D; 42 percent of African-American women of childbearing age are deficient in it; and more than 75 percent of pregnant women in the US are severely deficient in this crucial vitamin. Though appalling, these statistics are not surprising when you consider how sedentary and cloistered life has become. Some researchers claim that about 85 percent of the American population is vitamin D deficient.

<u>Vitamin D Prevents Cancer</u>: Did you know that there is a whole body of research that inversely correlates sunlight exposure (UV light) with breast, colon, rectal, prostate and ovarian cancer? There is no doubt either that Vitamin D is directly also correlated with your body's immune system. When it comes to immunity, this vitamin is observed to have an unusual ability to strengthen the body's innate immune response, which is a generalized response to potential harmful microbes. It is a non-specific, generic response unlike the adaptive immune system which 'remembers' pathogens and responds to them selectively.

In research published in the *Journal of Investigative Dermatology,* it was found that UV light stimulated a chemical in the skin which is a precursor to an anti-microbial peptide called LL-37. It is but logical that this amazing natural immune reaction takes place in the skin as the skin is a coat of armor or the body's first contact with all stimuli from the world outside. The skin is the largest organ in the body and it is the first line of defense before microbes penetrate other layers of defense. Another example of nature's supreme logic!

But how does Vitamin D actually work at the cellular level? When UV light strikes the skin, it interacts with a special type of cholesterol in the skin, and this cholesterol triggers the liver and kidney to convert Vitamin D into Vitamin D3. Vitamin D3 is the active form of Vitamin D and it promotes immune system function, controls cellular growth and absorbs calcium from the intestines.

Vitamin D3 can actually inhibit the growth of malignant melanoma, breast cancer, leukemia and breast tumors. It has also been shown to inhibit angiogenesis, which is the growth of new blood vessels that facilitate the spread of cancerous cells throughout the body.

Synthetic derivatives of Vitamin D3 have been found to halt the spread of breast cancer cells and cause regression of experimental mammary tumors. This is believed to be the case as Vitamin D and its derivatives are involved in regulating the expression of genes and protein products that prevent breast cancer.

Research has shown that some types of cancer cells contain Vitamin-D receptors, which make them susceptible to the anti-cancer effects of this vitamin-hormone or vitamin D3. Yes, this simple substance, abundantly present in your skin, is actually a tumor-suppressing hormone!

In 2007, the Canadian Cancer Society took a giant leap by promoting Vitamin D to prevent cancer though its national program.

But the American Cancer Society still refuses to acknowledge the enormous benefits of this natural chemical. And why would it? Acknowledging that the body is its best pharmacist would mean depriving pharma majors and radiologists of the billions of dollars they annually make off cancer.

Think about it. What are the two most oft-heard words associated with the cancer? 'Screening' and 'treatment'. Two simple words that the US government, doctors and Big Pharma promote for profit. Why on earth would the government and pharma companies shoot themselves in the foot by acknowledging that more than 75 percent of breast, colon, prostate and other types of cancer (the most common types) can be prevented, and possibly reversed, with Vitamin D?

This is mirrored in the hypocrisy of lobbies fighting a 'war against cancer'. The term reeks of profit and political motives and at the center of it all, not surprisingly, is the American Cancer Society (ACS). Research scholars who are experts on non-profit organizations have called the ACS the world's largest non-religious non-profit. Yet, according to some estimates, the organization spends less than 20 percent of its funds on services for cancer patients.

With funds received running into millions of dollars a year, this is an association that is actively *rooting* for cancer. Run like a high-tech corporation, the ACS has on its board some of the country's biggest honchos from the worlds of pharma, entertainment, film making and medical research. Funds pour in from the various corporate entities they run – news channels, pharma majors, film production studios etc – and are paid back to the outfits' honchos in six-figure salaries, field trips, fringe benefits, and overheads and salaries to run the ACS's numerous branches across the US.

Yet, the ACS goes down on bended knees every now and then pleading lack of funds to fight cancer, to solicit contributions from the public. There never was a bigger sham.

Only a small percentage of the ACS's funds are dedicated to cancer research, which predictably, is supportive of the pharma, biotech and related companies that bankroll the organization. So you see, the ACS, which also funds political campaigns and politicians, must keep cancer alive and kicking!

In modern medicine, regular screening, testing and radiotherapy are an inextricable part of cancer diagnosis and treatment. So apart from pharma companies who make some of the most toxic and most expensive cancer drugs, the ACS actively supports and promotes mammography and radiology manufacturers in a huge way, including manufacturers like Siemens, DuPont, General Electric, Eastman Kodak and Piker.

DuPont, ironically a global petrochemical manufacturer, is a major manufacturer of mammography machines. The company funds the ACS in a big way and serves on the organization's advisory boards and supports the ACS's awareness programs, an ideal platform to advertise its products and equipment. DuPont also sponsors TV programs and other media productions to promote mammography, and produces a host of promotional literature for medical facilities. How's that for a very profitable case of 'you scratch my back, I scratch yours'?

While on the subject of cancer and the approach conventional medicine takes to this disease, allow me to present my point of view. In my book, *Cancer Is Not A Disease – It's A Survival Mechanism*, I explain why cancer and other debilitating illnesses are not actual diseases but desperate and final attempts by the human body to stay alive for as long as circumstances permit.

It will perhaps astound you to learn that a person who is afflicted with the main causes of cancer (which constitute the real illness) would most likely die quickly unless he actually grew cancer cells. In the book, I provide evidence to this effect. Cancer will only occur after all other defense or healing mechanisms in the body have failed. In extreme circumstances, exposure to large amounts of cancer-producing agents (carcinogens) can bring about a collapse of the body's defenses within several weeks or months and allow for rapid and aggressive growth of a cancerous tumor. Usually, though, it takes many years, or even decades, for these so-called 'malignant' tumors to form.

Unfortunately, basic misconceptions or a complete lack of knowledge about the reasons behind tumor growth have turned 'malignant' tumors into vicious monsters that have no other purpose but to kill us in retaliation for our sins or for abusing the body. However, I am convinced that cancer is on our side, not against us. Unless we change our perception of what cancer really is, it will continue to resist healing, even through the best of treatments.

5. Nature's Pharmacy

Just like the body is its best doctor, Nature is the most abundantly-stocked pharmacy for the human species. Every single compound the body needs to heal and repair itself and, of course, to maintain good health, is naturally available.

There are hundreds of foods which have amazing healing-inducing properties. Many have immune-boosting properties while others are tumor-fighters. By not following Mother Nature's recipes, you're most likely to fall ill sooner or later. Read another way, this means that the greater the dependence on processed foods, the more likely you are to fall ill. Not only are you being deprived of natural nutrition but processed foods are full of chemical additives, which are harmful and also change the nature of the foods they are added to.

On the other hand, by eating from Nature's table, you may never fall ill in the first place. And if you fall ill now, in your search for a real cure to your ailment, you may discover that healthy food, fresh water and air, a peaceful disposition, good sleep, and a good amount of sunshine still constitute the best medicine you can find.

It would also stand you in good stead to eat according to your body type. This is because each body type reacts differently to the same food and requires different types of foods for optimal health. (For details on body types and superfoods, you can refer to my book, *Timeless Secrets of Rejuvenation and Health*)

6. Useful Tips On How To Deal With Infections Naturally

1. Acknowledge that you or your child have an infection and that the body and the germs involved are doing their best to restore its health and vitality. To support the body in this effort, we must ensure it has enough energy to cleanse, repair and heal itself. This can only happen if we allow the body to rest. Otherwise, we may use up all its energy, without which the healing will either stall or be slow.

2. Try to avoid medication. Drugs such as liquid paracetamol only suppress the body's healing response and lead to many more 'unrelated' physical and emotional problems in the future.

3. For a child, the period of illness is often a way to receive additional caring attention from his parents. He may get many extra cuddles, meals in bed, and stories at bedtime, etc. Of course, there may be parents who feel that their child's illness is very inconvenient and show their frustration by being harsh and insensitive to them. Sick children need and deserve special treatment and reassurance, especially when they are frightened or anxious.

4. A sick child should not be excited or stimulated by exposure to too much radio, television, or even visitors. Quiet activities such as reading to them, drawing, and board games help them to avoid dwelling on their illness too much. Make sure that they get extra sleep with early bedtimes, and daytime naps if they feel tired.

5. Sick children need to drink plenty of liquids to help remove toxins from the system. Warm water is the best drink for them and should be the first option; herb teas and freshly pressed, diluted carrot juice, and lemon or lime juice with some honey (avoid citrus juices if your child has mumps) can also be taken.

6. Avoid giving your child anything cold, such as cold beverages, ice cream, sugar, or sugar-containing foods; milk, yoghurt or other dairy products; meat, chicken, fish or any other form of protein food. As the child's digestive power is weakened during the illness, such foods will only putrefy and acidify the digestive system and further irritate the mucus lining. Sick children, like sick animals, generally do not want or need food. Fasting, while drinking only water, is the best way to encourage the body's healing response. When your child feels hungry, give him freshly cooked vegetable purées, soups, hot cereals like porridge/oatmeal with a little coconut sugar, or with good quality honey. Starving an infection is better than feeding it.

7. Children need to know what is happening to them during an illness and that it is going to pass soon. They also want reassurance that you are going to be there for them all the way.

8. If your child develops a fever, it is a sign of a healthy immune response. A raised temperature shows that the body has taken active charge of the situation and is fighting off an infection. Parents should remember that a high temperature does not necessarily mean that their child is very ill. As has been discovered recently, even a temperature of 41 degrees Celsius, or 106 degrees Fahrenheit, and slightly above is still not considered life-endangering. The most important thing to remember is that children and babies aged less than six months who are afflicted with fever need to drink plenty of water, as they tend to dehydrate quickly. Sponging them down with tepid water helps to keep the body more comfortable during this phase of healing. Expose and sponge only one part of the body at a time until it feels cool, then move on to the next one. Sponging the child's face and forehead also brings relief. And remember, fever stimulates the immune system, cleanses the body of toxins, turns up the heat high enough that the invading microbes cannot survive, creates more antibodies and white blood cells to help the body heal,

and walls off iron that bacteria feed on. Once the body has completed its work, the fever will drop naturally.

9. Another basic rule is to keep a chilly, feverish child warm and covered. This will make him sweat, particularly at night, and help to break the fever, which indicates that the body's 'fight' is nearly over. Hot, feverish children should be kept cool and occasionally be immersed in a bath of tepid water. If your child has accompanying symptoms such as itchy rashes, painful swollen glands, a cough or sore, sticky eyes, he is most likely to recover without any complications. In case he has any unusual symptoms, you may consult a natural practitioner of Ayurveda, Homeopathy, Chinese Medicine, etc, for home treatment remedies.

10. It is better not to give aspirin to children during an illness as this slows the fever response and interferes with the body's own healing. If your doctor insists on giving antibiotics to your child when he has one of the above illnesses or symptoms, try to find another doctor to give you a second opinion. Pau d' Arco, olive leaf extract, and exposure to sunlight (to make vitamin D) can act more effectively than antibiotics, without any side effects. In most cases, there is no need for drugs. In one large study published in 1987 in the British Medical Journal, 18,000 children received a homeopathic remedy against meningitis. None of the children got infected and not a single adverse effect developed from the treatment.

11. As a general precaution, do not take your child to daycare centers or nurseries too early. This can protect him from many childhood diseases. Daycare facilities increase the risk of Hib meningitis, for example, by 24 times. Many of the commercially run centers are frequently 'visited' by all sorts of bugs. The safest environment for a child in the first years of his life is his home.

12. Adults may benefit from a number of short sweat saunas or infrared saunas to help remove toxins faster.

13. Since toxins in the colon and liver always make it a lot more difficult for the body to heal, doing coffee enemas, water enemas, a Colema or colonic irrigation can quickly reduce severity of an infection or stop it altogether. (For more information on liver and colon cleansing methods, see Timeless Secrets of Health and Rejuvenation.) Constipation should be avoided by all means. Coffee enemas stimulate bile in the liver and help the liver remove toxins.

14. Immune strengthening herbs such as Pau D' Arco, olive leaf extract, Echinacea, golden seal, Astragalus and grapefruit seed extract may also be helpful. For topical infections, you may use raw

honey, bentonite clay, green clay, or urine packs (most effective). Elderberry has been used as a folk remedy for flu, colds, and coughs since the time of Hippocrates. And recently, an Israeli scientist discovered exactly why it works so well. In a controlled study that had flu sufferers recovering in record time, she found that elderberry literally 'disarms' viruses. The viruses simply were unable to penetrate the walls of the patients' cells.

15. Let an infection take its course, even if it takes a week or two, or longer. Stopping it can lead to repeat infections that become more severe each time. Remove toxins in the body instead, and the need for infection will die off naturally.

Chapter 10

Conclusion

After having read the data I have presented in this book, the next logical question is: if you don't immunize against disease, how do you safeguard your health?

If this book has opened a window in your mind even a little and you are able to see the vaccine game for what it truly is, the rest is easy. We usually assume that living healthy presupposes the absence of disease. Flip that around and you arrive at the following conclusion: 'The absence of disease lies in healthy living'. And therein, in that subtle semantic shift, lies an entire shift in the way you will perceive your life.

It would mean first identifying the sources of unhealthy living, and there are many! This would also imply a little soul-searching to identify lifestyle habits, and emotional and personality factors that contribute to ill-health and disease.

Not opting for vaccination also presupposes a firm belief in natural remedies, natural cures and a connection with the natural world. I am not advocating to a back-to-nature approach. That is not possible in the 21st century. However, most of us have come too far from our true nature and our evolutionary roots. Healing begins when you understand and accept this basic fact. (If you are interested, there is more on this subject in my book Timeless Secrets of Health and Rejuvenation)

At the risk of repeating myself, allow me to remind you that nature never intended that you pour chemical toxins into your body, for better or worse. Nature has created a wonderful natural pharmacy – within the human body and in the environment around.

Follow these principles and you automatically begin to strengthen your immune system. And that's your real armor against disease. When needed, alternative therapies are very beneficial as they reinforce the mind-body connection that is at the center of immunity, good health and disease.

But before I conclude, here's a glimpse at the future of vaccines, at least, the future as seen by vaccine researchers who love to wield their knives and scalpels. There are 145 additional vaccines being developed and tested in clinical trials, but thanks to the University of

California study on the lack of placebo disclosure during clinical trials, we now know how unscientific and fraudulent these trials can be.

Drug companies seek an ever-increasing predictable market in the US for these new vaccines, and we can expect that lobbyists will likely press the government for mandated use of many of them, both by children and adults. The following are a few examples of what is yet to come:

Stress Vaccine: And finally an answer to the scourge of modern living – a vaccine against stress. At least that's what Dr Robert Sapolsky of Stanford University is promising. Even more ironic: the proposed vaccine may use the herpes virus – a virus! – to carry genetically modified 'neuroprotective' genes into the depths of our brains to relieve us from chronic stress and produce a state of "focused calm".

Dr Sapolsky claimed in mid-2010 that these modified genes would help turn off the production of glucocorticoids, which build up in the body in states of prolonged stress. According to him, glucocorticoids play a crucial role in producing the 'fight or flight' response, which is essential to survival. But human beings have apparently lost the ability to turn them off. Hence, we need the help of a virus!

The good doctor has been researching his 'stress vaccine' for three decades and human trials are a long way off. But no doubt funding will pour in. Imagine the potential market for a product like this. No more wrestling with complex emotional states – those very things that make us human and allow us to learn and grow in confidence and wisdom. Just take a jab or pop a pill!

Syringes on Wings: Science is now toying with some pretty futuristic vaccine-delivery vehicles. And if these cutting-edge experiments are successful, the establishment may soon announce 'flying vaccines' and 'edible vaccines'.

Using a generous grant from the high-profile Bill and Melinda Gates Foundation in October 2008, a team of researchers from the Jichi Medical University in Japan are trying to turn mosquitoes into 'flying syringes' "so than when they bite human beings, they deliver vaccines".

While handing out endowments across the globe including the Japanese team, the foundation said it was looking "to fund research out of the realm of known scientific paradigms".

Snack On Them: The Japanese team is not the only group of scientists tampering with nature to restore us to good health. Scientists at Iowa State University are working on 'edible vaccines', by genetically modifying corn crops to deliver immunity to human beings who eat the corn as well as animals who feed on it.

This was reported in Meat And Poultry, a trade publication, in a May 5, 2009 article. The researchers propose to identify specific genes in specific pathogens (like the swine flu virus) which cause specific diseases and then incorporate these genes into the genotype of corn. Researchers hope this genetically-modified corn will contain the pathogen's genetic material in its genotype.

Experiments that try to introduce vaccines into the food chain (through food for human beings and animal feed) in this manner could raise serious ethical issues. Food manufacturers in the US, at least, have been able to work their way around transparency issues while labeling their products. As a result, consumers do not really know whether they are consuming GM foods or non-GM foods.

Two, there would be no way of telling what toxic genetic cocktails scientists may be introducing into innocuous-looking fruit and vegetables, and what exactly they are testing. Turning human beings into guinea pigs on their dinner table is nothing short of deception and unethical.

Imagine eating your vaccines from a giant bag of corn chips or your breakfast cereal in a bowl of milk! Vaccination via processed foods would place your life in double jeopardy. What next?

Robot Antibodies: Next on the cutting edge of the vaccine laboratory table are artificial antibodies. Scientists at Emory University at Atlanta have created an artificial antibody to target cancerous tumors with the help of another cutting-edge bio-tool: the nanoparticle.

Antibodies are large and cannot reach the recesses of a tumor. In January 2009, scientists at Emory University announced that they had overcome this hurdle by creating a synthetic antibody that was less than 20 percent the size of the natural antibody. Next, they found a way to bind their artificial antibody to a nanoparticle. This dual-weapon was then used to target cancerous tumors in mice.

How does this work? Antibodies are agents produced in response to an infection or pathogenic process in the human body. Many of them are specific as they are linked to a specific disease such as cancer. In this case, scientists fabricated an artificial anti-EGFR (epidermal growth factor receptor) antibody which would home in on the tumor and could this be used as an effective vehicle to carry a nanoparticle. This technique could also be used for diagnostic and therapeutic purposes, the scientists say.

Nanoparticles show up on an MRI (Magnetic Resonance Imaging) scan and are regarded as valuable diagnostic tools. They can also be used to carry drugs and are hence regarded as efficient therapeutic carriers.

So, armed with a vehicle that goes where none like it have gone before (artificial antibody) and a drug carrier (nanoparticle), scientists believe they could use this new technology in the diagnosis and treatment of cancer.

Antibodies are the antithesis of antigens or the active viral agent in a vaccine. If researchers can manufacture an artificial antibody for tumors, using the technology for vaccines may be the next logical step.

Medical wizardry can be irresistibly seductive. But make no mistake. The more you tamper with the natural order of things, the greater the repercussions on your body. Genetic manipulation is injurious to your health!

I would like to encourage you to join the National Vaccine Information Center (NVIC) to help protect the right to informed consent to vaccination. NVIC wants to help you, their members, to organize and make a difference in your home state (in the US only) right where you live to protect and expand vaccine exemptions. It is at the state level that mass vaccination policies are made, and it is at the state level where your action to protect your rights can have the greatest impact. Also, when national vaccine issues occur, you will be plugged in to the information and action items necessary to make sure your voice is heard.

Web site: www.nvicadvocacy.org
Facebook: www.facebook.com/national.vaccine

References and Resources

http://74.125.153.132/search?q=cache:3GII2dgd6OOJ:www.whale.to/vaccine

http://pediatrics.aappublications.org/cgi/content/full/112/6/1394

http://www.quackwatch.com/03HealthPromotion/immu/immu00.html

http://www.mad-cow.org/

http://www.mad-cow.org/00/may00_news.html

http://www.mad-cow.org/00/01jan_news.html

http://www.emedicinehealth.com/mad_cow_disease

http://www.ncbi.nlm.nih.gov/pubmed/20067537

http://74.125.153.132/search?q=cache:k6kLlng7n88J:www.anellomedicalwriting.com/SV40-%2520HMS%2520Beagle.doc+SV40+controversy&cd=1&hl=en&ct=clnk&gl=in

http://74.125.153.132/search?q=cache:5ZF6EiORIEoJ:www.hpakids.org/holistic-health/articles/122/1/Smallpox-Vaccine:-Does-it-Work%253F+smallpox+england+1871&cd=4&hl=en&ct=clnk&gl=in

http://74.125.153.132/search?q=cache:YBgSr8dRdUcJ:en.wikipedia.org/wiki/Cowpox+cowpox+vaccina&cd=1&hl=en&ct=clnk&gl=in

http://tropej.oxfordjournals.org/cgi/pdf_extract/21/supp1/51

http://www.sourcewatch.org/index.php?title=Pharmaceutical_industry#Dr._Jonas_Salk_senate_hearings_.26_VAPP

http://www.soilandhealth.org/02/0201hyglibcat/020132sinclair/vaccinaion.htm

http://www.vaccineinformation.org/measles/qandavax.asp

http://www.drellegee.com/vaccination.html

http://74.125.153.132/search?q=cache:MD5zaUYtQH0J:www.sv40foundation.org/+sv40&cd=3&hl=en&ct=clnk&gl=in

http://www.sv40foundation.org/SV40-from-PV.html

http://www.childbirthsolutions.com/articles/postpartum/dispelling2/index.php

http://www.scidev.net/en/health/clinical-ethics/nigeria-sues-pfizer-over-drug

http://www.childbirthsolutions.com/articles/postpartum/dispelling/index.php

http://www.naturalnews.com/022400_vaccines
http://vaers.hhs.gov/data
http://www.childbirthsolutions.com/articles/postpartum/dispel
ling/index.php
http://www.naturalnews.com/022400_vaccines
http://www.whale.to/vaccine
http://www.jabs.org.uk/forum/topic.asp?TOPIC_ID=1391
http://educate-
yourself.org/vcd/howensteinwhyyoushouldavoidvaccines03feb0
7.shtml
http://articles.mercola.com/sites/articles/archive/2004/05/12/
vaccination-dangers.aspx
http://www.absoluteastronomy.com/topics/Vaccination
http://www.naturalnews.com/polio.html
http://www.naturalnews.com/021572.html
http://www.naturalnews.com/022400_vaccines
http://www.naturalnews.com/026951_vaccination_polio_immun
e
http://www.vaclib.org/basic/manu.htm
http://www.msnbc.msn.com/id/21034344/ns/health-
infectious_diseases/
http://www.naturalnews.com/026951_vaccination_polio_immun
e
http://www.aldara1.com/Overview%20&%20Summaries/immu
ne
http://www.naturalnews.com/026951_vaccination_polio_immun
e
http://www.naturalnews.com/026951_vaccination_polio_immun
e
http://www.google.co.in/#hl=en&source=hp&q=nigeria+polio+o
utbreak&btnG=Google+Search&meta=&aq=0&oq=nigeria+polio+
out&fp=31fb0df7a2e827f9
http://www.msnbc.msn.com/id/21149823/
http://www.washingtonpost.com/wp-
dyn/content/article/2007/10/05/AR2007100501193.html
http://news.bbc.co.uk/2/hi/2070634.stm
http://www.naturalnews.com/022508_polio_measles_immunizat
ion
http://www.naturalnews.com/022382_disease
http://www.naturalnews.com/022572_vaccines

http://www.vanityfair.com/politics/features/2011/01/deadly-medicine
http://www.naturalnews.com/021572.html
http://www.naturalnews.com/HPV_vaccine
http://www.naturalnews.com/027218_health_vaccines
http://www.naturalnews.com/027017_HPV_HPV_vaccine
http://www.naturalnews.com/026463_HPV_vaccine
http://www.naturalnews.com/026019_HPV_HPV_vaccine
http://www.naturalnews.com/025411_HPV_allergic
http://www.naturalnews.com/027196_cancer_cervical_cancer_cancer_vaccine
http://www.naturalnews.com/026951_vaccination_polio_immune
http://www.whale.to/a/nkuba.htm
http://educate-yourself.org/cn/vaccinationsinUganda22dec03.shtml
http://www.google.co.in/#hl=en&source=hp&q=nigeria+polio+outbreak&btnG=Google+Search&meta=&aq=0&oq=nigeria+polio+out&fp=31fb0df7a2e827f9
http://www.msnbc.msn.com/id/21149823/
http://www.washingtonpost.com/wp-dyn/content/article/2007/10/05/AR2007100501193.html
http://news.bbc.co.uk/2/hi/2070634.stm
http://articles.mercola.com/sites/articles/archive/2009/12/01/Polio-Vaccine-Blamed-for-Outbreaks-in-Nigeria
http://74.125.153.132/search?q=cache:cB60wEgl_JYJ:www.pbs.org/newshour/updates/health/july-dec09/polio_08-24.html+nigeria+polio+outbreak&cd=2&hl=en&ct=clnk&gl=in
http://www.naturalnews.com/027365_flu
http://www.fightbackh1n1.com/2009/08/criminal-chargesanzeigen.html
http://www.vaclib.org/basic/manu.htm
http://www.whale.to/vaccine
http://www.timesonline.co.uk/tol/news/science
http://www.naturalnews.com/027248_disease
http://www.naturalnews.com/027248_disease
http://www.naturalnews.com/chronic_fatigue.html
http://www.naturalnews.com/024788_chronic_fatigue_chronic_fatigue_syndrome_candida.html
http://www.microbiologybytes.com/virology/Retroviruses.html

http://answers.yahoo.com/question/index?qid=2008061203011
0AAC2ixe
http://www.google.co.in/search?hl=en&q=cfs+virus=
http://www.ehow.com/how-does_5499473_diseases-caused-
retrovirus.html
http://www.scientificamerican.com/article.cfm?id=chronic-
fatigue-syndrome-retrovirus
http://www.nhs.uk/news/2010/01January/Pages/Virus-link-to-
CFS-in-doubt.aspx
http://www.allnaturalinfo.com/medical_danger.htm
http://www.naturalnews.com/024004_cancer_vaccines
http://www.whale.to/vaccines
http://www.drlenhorowitz.com/news/vaccine
http://educate-
yourself.org/vcd/howensteinwhyyoushouldavoidvaccines03feb0
7.shtml
http://www.vaclib.org/basic/manu.htm
http://news.bbc.co.uk/2/hi/health/8493753.stm
http://news.bbc.co.uk/2/hi/health/8483865.stm
http://news.bbc.co.uk/2/hi/health/8481583.stm
http://news.bbc.co.uk/2/hi/health/6289166.stm
http://news.bbc.co.uk/2/hi/health/1808956.stm
http://www.naturalnews.com/026434_vaccines
http://www.naturalnews.com/022400_vaccines
http://www.naturalnews.com/026951_vaccination_polio_immun
e
http://www.naturalnews.com/027483_SIGA_Technologies_vacci
nes
http://www.reuters.com/article/scienceNews/idUSTRE5AF5EO
20091117
http://articles.mercola.com/sites/articles/archive/2009/11/07/
Beware-of-the-New-Useless-and-Dangerous-Vaccines-in-the-
Works.aspx
http://articles.mercola.com/sites/articles/archive/2009/11/14/
Expert-Pediatrician-Exposes-Vaccine-Myths.aspx
http://www.soilandhealth.org/02/0201hyglibcat/020132sinclai
r/vaccinaion.htm
http://www.whale.to/vaccines
http://www.whale.to/vaccine
http://www.childbirthsolutions.com/articles/postpartum/dispel
ling/index.php

http://www.childbirthsolutions.com/articles/postpartum/dispel
ling2/index.php
http://vaers.hhs.gov/data
http://www.timesonline.co.uk/tol/news/science
http://www.allnaturalinfo.com/medical_danger.htm
http://74.125.153.132/search?q=cache:xh-
k55OsM2UJ:homeopathyworldcommunity.ning.com/forum/topic
s/expose-on-the-true-nature-
of+Communicable+Diseases+Handbook+bennett+searle&cd=9&h
l=en&ct=clnk&gl=in
http://www.absoluteastronomy.com/topics/Vaccination_and_rel
igion
http://www.naturalnews.com/022508_polio_measles_immunizat
ion
http://www.naturalnews.com/022382_disease
http://www.naturalnews.com/022572_vaccines
http://www.vaccinationdebate.com/web1.html
http://www.drellegee.com/vaccination.html
http://www.vaccinationdebate.com/
http://www.naturalnews.com/027258_vaccines
http://www.timesonline.co.uk/tol/news/science
http://www.soilandhealth.org/02/0201hyglibcat/020132sinclai
r/vaccinaion.htm
http://www.naturalnews.com/polio.html
http://www.whale.to/a/vaccination_quote_banners.html
http://educate-
yourself.org/vcd/howensteinwhyyoushouldavoidvaccines03feb0
7.shtml
http://www.naturalnews.com/026434_vaccines
http://www.healthfreedomusa.org/?p=448
http://www.drlenhorowitz.com/news/vaccine
http://articles.mercola.com/sites/articles/archive/2009/12/01/
Polio-Vaccine-Blamed-for-Outbreaks-in-Nigeria
http://www.theecologist.org/pages/a...
http://www.theecologist.org/pages/a...
http://www.whale.to/v/salk6.html   .
http://www.naturalnews.com/026434_vaccines
http://articles.mercola.com/sites/articles/archive/2010/02/09/
6-principles-you-should-know-before-making-an-informed-
swine-flu

http://www.naturalnews.com/026934_health_public_health_qua
rantine.html
http://www.prisonplanet.com/europeans-reject-swine-flu
http://www.naturalnews.com/026951_vaccination_polio_immun
e
http://www.naturalnews.com/027222_swine_flu
http://www.naturalnews.com/vaccinations.html
http://www.naturalnews.com/026907_food_vaccination_health.h
tml
http://www.naturalnews.com/026562_vaccinations_NaturalNew
s_The_Constitution.html
http://www.naturalnews.com/026538_vaccination_vaccinations_
Chi.html
http://www.naturalnews.com/026227_vaccines
http://www.naturalnews.com/025608_health_economic_stimulu
s_bill_economic_stimulus.html
http://www.naturalnews.com/026934_health_public_health_qua
rantine.html
http://www.naturalnews.com/027597_medical_mafia_medicine
http://www.naturalnews.com/024779_HPV_cancer_vaccination.
html
http://www.naturalnews.com/disease
http://www.rense.com/general86/fluu.htm
http://www.naturalnews.com/026434_vaccines
http://www.whale.to/b/mullins2.html
http://www.prisonplanet.com/europeans-reject-swine-flu
http://www.progressiveconvergence.c...
http://www.americanchronicle.com/ar...
http://healthfreedoms.org/2009/11/1...
http://www.theforbiddenknowledge.com/hardtruth/patriot_act.
htm
http://en.wikipedia.org/wiki/Model_State_Emergency_Health_Po
wers_Act
http://74.125.153.132/search?q=cache%3AFq086GI6tVEJ%3Aw
ww.turningpointprogram.org%2FPages%2Fpdfs%2Fstatute_mod
%2Fphsm_fact_sheet_emerg_health_powers_act.pdf+Model+State
+Emergency+Health+Powers+Act&hl=en&gl=in
http://www.vaccinationeducation.com/hepatitis.html
http://www.healing-arts.org/children
http://www.gulfwarvets.com/hep-b.htm

http://74.125.153.132/search?q=cache:IBWYQmbko2wJ:www.w
hale.to/v/horowitz.html+france+hepatitis+g+deaths
http://en.wikipedia.org/wiki/Contaminated_haemophilia_blood_
products
http://www.eugenics-watch.com/roots/chap12.html
http://www.naturalnews.com/026434_vaccines
http://birdflu666.wordpress.com/2009/07/09/who-has-the-
power-to-order-forced-vaccines
http://loveforlife.com.au/content/09/07/14/french-doctor
http://www.nvic.org/vaccine
http://www.naturalnews.com/vaccinations.html
http://www.naturalnews.com/law_enforcement.html
http://74.125.153.132/search?q=cache:pzSa5OKuhxoJ:www.plu.
edu/~goffdl/doc/vaccination.doc+new+jersey+compulsory+vacc
ination+2007&cd=5&hl=en&ct=clnk&gl=in
http://www.namiscc.org/News/2003/Spring/ChildMedicationSa
fetyAct.htm
http://content.nejm.org/cgi/content/full/360/19/1981
http://vaccineawakening.blogspot.com/2007/11/police-with-
dogs-vaccinating-kids-in.html
http://www.aapsonline.org/press/nr-11-16-07.php
http://www.naturalnews.com/Abraham_Cherrix.html
http://blog.nj.com/jerseyblogs/2007/12/njs_new_vaccine
http://www.nytimes.com/2009/01/04/nyregion/new-
jersey/04flunj.html?ref=education
http://74.125.153.132/search?q=cache:0MOqQ3omisMJ:www.inj
uryboard.com/national-news/flu
http://www.disinfo.com/2007/12/help-stop-forced-vaccination-
of-children
http://irdial.com/blogdial/?p=2114
http://curezone.com/forums/fm.asp?i=1489548
http://blog.nj.com/jerseyblogs/2007/12/njs_new_vaccine
http://74.125.153.132/search?q=cache:SaZpXwpFZoOJ:www.nat
uralnews.com/026934_health_public_health_quarantine.html+for
ced+vaccination+us&cd=1&hl=en&ct=clnk&gl=in
http://www.fightbackh1n1.com/2009/10/massachusetts-house-
of-representatives.html
http://veglawyer.wordpress.com/2007/11/20/parents-shots-or-
slammer/
http://www.naturalnews.com/022267.html
http://www.csmonitor.com/2007/1119/p02s04-ussc.html

http://vaccineawakening.blogspot.com/2007/11/police-with-dogs-vaccinating-kids-in.html

http://www.google.co.in/#hl=en&source=hp&q=maryland+forced+vaccination&meta=&aq=7m&aqi=g6g-m4&aql=&oq=forced+vacc&gs_rfai=&fp=cc92a28a1a68ec6a

http://blogs.myspace.com/index.cfm?fuseaction=blog.view&friendID=207506724&blogID=330335859&Mytoken=1F0E28E1-7A16-432C-B7F426C5582B40D415028805

http://www.thenhf.com/vaccinations/vac_299.htm

http://www.namiscc.org/News/2003/Spring/ChildMedicationSafetyAct.htm

http://www.naturalnews.com/026735_health_vaccination_CODEX.html

http://www.naturalnews.com/027106_vaccination_Vitamin_D_vaccinations.html

http://www.naturalnews.com/026562_vaccinations_NaturalNews_The_Constitution.html

http://www.naturalnews.com/026538_vaccination_vaccinations_Chi.html

http://www.naturalnews.com/026227_vaccines

http://www.chron.com/disp/story.mpl/nb/bellaire/news/6387161.html

http://www.naturalnews.com/026227_vaccines

http://www.naturalnews.com/024575_health_hospital_doctors

http://www.naturalnews.com/024779_HPV_cancer_vaccination.html

http://www.globalresearch.ca/index.php?context=va&aid=14433

http://www.semp.us/publications/biot_reader.php?BiotID=177

http://www.naturalnews.com/023133_health_New_York_medicine

http://www.whale.to/vaccine

http://www.youtube.com/watch?v=MK2rkReq28A

http://afp.google.com/article/ALeqM5i4hpnz5eOMpxfld81tEZYsC23teg

http://www.conspiracyplanet.com/channel.cfm?channelid=8&contentid=5964

http://www4.dr-rath-foundation.org/open_letters/pharma_laws_history.html#rockefeller

http://www.whale.to/vaccine

http://www.whale.to/a/gates1.html
http://lists.essential.org/pipermail/ip-health/2002-May/003052.html
http://www.latimes.com/news/nationworld/nation/la-na-gatesx07jan07,0,6827615.story?coll=la-home-headlines
http://www.conspiracyplanet.com/channel.cfm?channelid=8&contentid=6746
http://afp.google.com/article/ALeqM5i4hpnz5eOMpxfld81tEZYsC23teg
http://www.becomehealthynow.com/article/bodyimmune/1142
http://www.neurope.eu/articles/97835.php
http://www.naturalnews.com/027222_swine_flu
http://www.vierascheibner.org/index.php?view=article&catid=52%3Ageneral-essays-by-viera&id=80%3Areview-of-vaccination-by-viera-scheibner-irene-alleger&option=com_content&Itemid=63
http://www.naturalnews.com/chronic_fatigue.html
http://www.google.co.in/#hl=en&source=hp&q=vaccine
http://chronicfatigue.about.com/od/whatischronicfatigue/a/what_is_CFS.htm
http://www.ncbi.nlm.nih.gov/pubmed/17364497
http://chetday.com/janecfids.html
http://www.whale.to/vaccines
http://www.immune
http://www.immune
http://www.anapsid.org/cnd/diffdx/polio2.html
http://www.whale.to/w/douglas.html
http://www.sleepydust.net/polio-vaccine
http://www.ei-resource.org/articles/gulf-war-syndrome-articles/how-vaccinations-work/
http://autismfacts.com/services.php?page_id=188
http://www.healing-arts.org/children
http://chetday.com/hepbarticle.html
http://www.whale.to/vaccine
http://www.thinktwice.com/hepb.htm
http://www.scribd.com/doc/24410018/Hepatitis-b-Vaccine
http://www.scribd.com/doc/24410018/Hepatitis-b-Vaccine#fullscreen:on
http://www.pslgroup.com/dg/bf712.htm
http://www.whale.to/a/spalding.html
http://www.naturodoc.com/library/bio-war/HepB.htm

http://autismfacts.com/services.php?page_id=188
http://articles.mercola.com/sites/articles/archive/2010/04/17/
major-vaccine
http://www.naturalnews.com/HPV_vaccines
http://www.naturalnews.com/cancer_vaccine
http://www.naturalnews.com/027196_cancer_cervical_cancer_ca
ncer_vaccine
http://www.i-sis.org.uk/HPV_Vaccine_Controversy.php
http://www.newswithviews.com/NWV-News/news57.htm
http://cancer.about.com/od/hpvcervicalcancervaccine/a/contro
versyHPV.htm
http://anthraxvaccine.blogspot.com/2010/03/gardasil-49-us-
deaths
http://www.thenhf.com/vaccinations/vaccinations_183.htm
http://jeannehannah.typepad.com/blog_jeanne_hannah_traver/g
ardasil/
http://www.24-7-news.com/archives/4021
http://www.wsws.org/articles/2004/nov2004/viox-n22.shtml
http://www.msnbc.msn.com/id/6192603/
http://www.naturalnews.com/027582_Merck_Vioxx.html
http://www.naturalnews.com/028143_children
http://www.naturalnews.com/028686_Big_Pharma
http://articles.mercola.com/sites/articles/archive/2010/03/09/
airlines-finally-recognize-its-persons-immune
http://www.naturalnews.com/022508_polio_measles_immunizat
ion
http://www.naturalnews.com/027203_vaccination_health_vacci
nes
http://educate-
yourself.org/vcd/howensteinwhyyoushouldavoidvaccines03feb0
7.shtml
http://articles.mercola.com/sites/articles/archive/2010/03/30/
central-figure-in-vaccine
http://articles.mercola.com/sites/articles/archive/2009/10/20/
Mild-Swine-Flu-and-Over-Hyped-Vaccine.aspx
http://www.know-vaccines
http://www.whale.to/vaccine
http://www.know-vaccines
http://autismfacts.com/services.php?page_id=188
http://www.healing-arts.org/children
http://www.safeminds.org/

http://www.huffingtonpost.com/david-kirby/autism
http://www.healing-arts.org/children
http://www.nytimes.com/2002/11/10/magazine/the-not-so-crackpot-autism
http://www.whale.to/a/blaylock.html#The_neurotoxicity_of_aluminium_
http://www.huffingtonpost.com/robert-f-kennedy-jr/time-for-cdc-to-come-clea_b_16550.html
http://articles.mercola.com/sites/articles/archive/2004/09/22/blaylock-vaccine
http://articles.mercola.com/sites/articles/archive/2005/07/23/mercury-vaccines
http://www.whale.to/vaccine
http://www.whale.to/vaccine
http://www.whale.to/a/blaylock.html
http://en.wikipedia.org/wiki/2000_Simpsonwood_CDC_conference
http://www.naturalnews.com/011764.html
http://www.whale.to/vaccine
http://www.naturalnews.com/011764.html
http://www.time.com/time/health/article/0,8599,1721109,00.html
http://autismfacts.com/services.php?page_id=206
http://www.ageofautism.com/2008/05/autism
http://weblogs.baltimoresun.com/news/opinion/2009/06/the_vaccineautism_controversy.html
http://www.naturalnews.com/027178_vaccines
http://www.naturalnews.com/027119_hepatitis_B_hepatitis_autism
http://www.naturalnews.com/026827_autism
http://www.naturalnews.com/027178_vaccines
http://www.naturalnews.com/027175_vaccines
http://www.youtube.com/watch?v=MK2rkReq28A
http://www.youtube.com/watch?v=_Ck3GLASVTA&NR=1
http://www.youtube.com/watch?v=dxxYIeE0_p0&feature=related
http://www.aapsonline.org/testimony/emerpind.htm
http://en.wikipedia.org/wiki/USA_PATRIOT_Act

About Andreas Moritz

Andreas Moritz (born January 27, 1954), an American writer born and raised in Southwest Germany, is also a lecturer of Ayurveda, integrative medicine, and mind, body and spirit. He has also specialized in creating fine art as a healing modality. Moritz began his career in Europe as an iridologist (science of eye interpretation) with special focus on identifying and addressing the root causes of illness. He is a former leader of the Transcendental Meditation ('TM') movement. In the mid-1990s, he began publishing self-help books on alternative medicine and mind/body/spirit integration.

Early life, education and accomplishments

From age six, Andreas Moritz had to deal with a number of severe illnesses (e.g., juvenile arthritis, arrhythmia, anemia, frequent bouts of passing out [fainting] and irritable bowel syndrome [IBS]). Although his main fields of interest were architecture, music and athletics, he had no choice but to spend the majority of his childhood trying to understand why he was so ill. Accordingly, at age 12, Moritz began studying diet, nutrition and various approaches to natural healing and well-being. In 1970, Moritz began to practice the Transcendental Meditation technique (TM) and Yoga which put an end to his abnormally low blood pressure and regular fainting spells. By age 19, Moritz had fully restored his own health without traditional medicine or outside intervention.

After completing 14 years of primary and higher education in Aalen – a picturesque town in Southwest Germany – Moritz received his 'Abitur' degree at the Schubert Gymnasium, qualifying him to enter university for advanced academic study. In 1974, Moritz completed his seven-month Teacher Training Course, becoming qualified as a teacher of the Transcendental Meditation ('TM') technique. He taught meditation to thousands of people around the world over a span of 20 years.

In 1980, after completing his iridology training with his uncle, Dr. Harry Kirchofer, a leading iridology physician and naturopath in Germany in his time (1914–1996), Moritz proceeded to study and perform research on mind/body medicine at Maharishi European Research University (MERU) in Seelisberg, Switzerland.

In 1981, as part of his training at MERU, Moritz began his studies of Ayurvedic medicine. To learn from some of the world's most renowned physicians of Ayurveda, including Dr. V. M. Dwivedi, Dr. Balraj Maharishi and Dr. Brihaspati Dev Triguna, Moritz travelled to New Delhi, India (1981–1982). From 1982–1983 Moritz introduced heads of state and members of governments in Ethiopia and Kenya to more holistic and cost effective approaches to healthcare than were available in these impoverished African countries at the time.

In 1991, Moritz finalized his Ayurveda training and qualified as a practitioner of Ayurveda (vaidya) in New Zealand.

Moritz lived on the island of Cyprus from 1985–1998, from where he travelled around the world, personally lecturing on and providing alternative healing modalities to governmental leaders who had fallen seriously ill, including the late Prime Minister of Greece, Andreas Papandreou.

Rather than being satisfied with merely treating the symptoms of illness, which typically causes harmful side effects, Moritz dedicated his life's work to understanding and effectively dealing with the root causes of illness, thereby allowing the body to naturally heal itself.

In 1988, Moritz studied and graduated in the Japanese healing art of shiatsu at the British School of Shiatsu in London, England, which has given him insights into the energy systems of the body.

In 1998, Moritz immigrated to Minnesota, in the United States, where he married and began to offer his services to the American people.

As of December 2010, Andreas Moritz is also the author of 13 books, many of which have been translated into several foreign languages, including Russian, Spanish, Chinese, German, Japanese, Greek, Portuguese, French, Dutch and Italian. These include: Timeless Secrets of Health and Rejuvenation, The Amazing Liver and Gallbladder Flush, Cancer Is Not a Disease! — It's A Survival Mechanism, Lifting the Veil of Duality, It's Time to Come Alive, Heart Disease No More!, Simple Steps to Total Health, Diabetes–No More!, Ending the AIDS Myth, Heal Yourself with Sunlight, Feel Great, Lose Weight, and Hear The Whispers–Live Your Dream.

Health and wellness topics, recorded by iHealth-Tube and made available at his web site, www.ener-chi.com. For several years, Andreas ran a free forum 'Ask Andreas Moritz' on the large health website, where over four million readers have read or commented on his messages.

Since taking up residence in the United States in 1998, Andreas has been involved in developing a new and innovative system of healing – called Ener-Chi Art™ – which targets root causes of many chronic illnesses. Ener-Chi Art consists of a series of light ray-encoded oil paintings that can instantly restore vital energy flow (Chi) in the organs and systems of the body. Andreas is also the founder of Sacred Santémony – a powerful system of specially generated frequencies of sound and energy that can transform deep-seated fears, allergies, traumas and mental or emotional blocks into useful opportunities for growth and inspiration within a matter of minutes.

Other books by Andreas Moritz

The Amazing Liver and Gallbladder Flush
A Powerful Do-It-Yourself Tool
to Optimize Your Health and Wellbeing

In this revised edition of his bestselling book, *The Amazing Liver Cleanse*, Andreas Moritz addresses the most common but rarely recognized cause of illness - gallstones congesting the liver. Although those who suffer an excruciatingly painful gallbladder attack are clearly aware of the stones congesting this vital organ, few people realize that hundreds if not thousands of gallstones (mainly clumps of hardened bile) have accumulated in their liver, often causing no pain or symptoms for decades.

Most adults living in the industrialized world, and especially those suffering a chronic illness such as heart disease, arthritis, MS, cancer, or diabetes, have gallstones blocking the bile ducts of their liver. Furthermore, 20 million Americans suffer from gallbladder attacks every year. In many cases, treatment consists merely of removing the gallbladder, at the cost of $5 billion a year. This purely symptom-oriented approach, however, does not eliminate the cause of the illness, and in many cases, sets the stage for even more serious conditions.

This book provides a thorough understanding of what causes gallstones in both the liver and gallbladder and explains why these stones can be held responsible for the most common diseases so prevalent in the world today. It provides the reader with the knowledge needed to recognize the stones and gives the necessary, do-it-yourself instructions to remove them painlessly in the comfort of one's own home. The book also shares practical guidelines on how to prevent new gallstones from forming. The widespread success of *The Amazing Liver & Gallbladder Flush* stands as a testimony to the strength and effectiveness of the cleanse itself. This powerful yet simple cleanse has led to extraordinary improvements in health and wellness among thousands of people who have already given themselves the precious gift of a strong, clean, revitalized liver.

Timeless Secrets of
Health and Rejuvenation
Breakthrough Medicine for the 21st Century
(550 pages, 8 ½ x 11 inches)

This book meets the increasing demand for a clear and comprehensive guide that can helps people to become self-sufficient regarding their health and wellbeing. It answers some of the most pressing questions of our time: How does illness arise? Who heals, and who doesn't? Are we destined to be sick? What causes aging? Is it reversible? What are the major causes of disease, and how can we eliminate them? What simple and effective practices can I incorporate into my daily routine that will dramatically improve my health?

Topics include: The placebo effect and the mind/body mystery; the laws of illness and health; the four most common risk factors for disease; digestive disorders and their effects on the rest of the body; the wonders of our biological rhythms and how to restore them if disrupted; how to create a life of balance; why to choose a vegetarian diet; cleansing the liver gallbladder, kidneys and colon; removing allergies; giving up smoking, naturally; using sunlight as medicine; the 'new' causes of heart disease, cancer, diabetes, and AIDS; and a scrutinizing look at antibiotics, blood transfusions, ultrasound scans, and immunization programs.

Timeless Secrets of Health and Rejuvenation sheds light on all major issues of healthcare and reveals that most medical treatments, including surgery, blood transfusions, and pharmaceutical drugs, are avoidable when certain key functions in the body are restored through the natural methods described in the book. The reader also learns about the potential dangers of medical diagnosis and treatment, as well as the reasons vitamin supplements, 'health foods', low-fat products, 'wholesome' breakfast cereals, diet foods, and diet programs may have contributed to the current health crisis rather than helped to resolve it. The book includes a complete program of healthcare, which is primarily based on the ancient medical system of Ayurveda and the vast amount of personal experience Andreas Moritz has gained in the field of health restoration during the past 37 years.

Cancer is Not a Disease!
It's A Survival Mechanism
Discover Cancer's Hidden Purpose, Heal its Root Causes, and be Healthier Than Ever!

In *Cancer is Not a Disease,* Andreas Moritz proves the point that cancer is the physical symptom that reflects our body's final attempt to deal with life-threatening cell congestion and toxins. He claims that removing the underlying conditions that force the body to produce cancerous cells, sets the preconditions for complete healing of our body, mind, and emotions.

This book confronts you with a radically new understanding of cancer – one that revolutionized the current cancer model. On the average, today's conventional 'treatments' of killing, cutting out, or burning cancerous cells offer most patients a remission rate of a mere 7 percent, and the majority of these survivors are 'cured' for just five years or fewer. Prominent cancer researcher and professor at the University of California at Berkeley, Dr. Hardin Jones, stated: "Patients are as well, or better off, untreated..." Any published success figures in cancer survival statistics are offset by equal or better scores among those receiving no treatment at all. More people are killed by cancer treatments than are saved by them.

Cancer is Not a Disease shows you why traditional cancer treatments are often fatal, what actually causes cancer, and how you can remove the obstacles that prevent the body from healing itself. Cancer is not an attempt on your life; on the contrary, this 'dread disease' is the body's final, desperate effort to save your life. Unless we change our perception of what cancer really is, it will continue to threaten the life of nearly one out of every two people. This book opens a door for those who wish to turn feelings of victimhood into empowerment and self-mastery, and disease into health.

Topics of the book include:

- Reasons why the body is forced to develop cancer cells
- How to identify and remove the causes of cancer
- Why most cancers disappear by themselves, without medical intervention
- Why radiation, chemotherapy, and surgery never cure cancer

- Why some people survive cancer despite undergoing dangerously radical treatments
- The roles of fear, frustration, low self-worth, and repressed anger in the origination of cancer
- How to turn self-destructive emotions into energies that promote health and vitality
- Spiritual lessons behind cancer

Lifting the Veil of Duality
Your Guide to Living without Judgment

"Do you know that there is a place inside you - hidden beneath the appearance of thoughts, feelings, and emotions - that does not know the difference between good and evil, right and wrong, light and dark? From that place you embrace the opposite values of life as One. In this sacred place you are at peace with yourself and at peace with your world." - Andreas Moritz

In Lifting the Veil of Duality, Andreas Moritz poignantly exposes the illusion of duality. He outlines a simple way to remove every limitation that you have imposed upon yourself during the course of living in the realm of duality. You will be prompted to see yourself and the world through a new lens – the lens of clarity, discernment, and non-judgment. You will also discover that mistakes, accidents, coincidences, negativity, deception, injustice, wars, crime, and terrorism all have a deeper purpose and meaning in the larger scheme of things. So naturally, much of what you will read may conflict with the beliefs you currently hold. Yet you are not asked to change your beliefs or opinions. Instead, you are asked to have an open mind, for only an open mind can enjoy freedom from judgment.

Our personal views and worldviews are currently challenged by a crisis of identity. Some are being shattered altogether. The collapse of our current world order forces humanity to deal with the most basic issues of existence. You can no longer avoid taking responsibility for the things that happen to you. When you do accept responsibility, you also empower and heal yourself.

Lifting the Veil of Duality shows you how you create or subdue your ability to fulfill your desires. Furthermore, you will find intriguing explanations about the mystery of time, the truth and illusion of reincarnation, the oftentimes misunderstood value of prayer, what makes relationships work, and why so often they don't. Find out why injustice is an illusion that has managed to haunt us throughout the ages. Learn about our original separation from the Source of life and what this means with regard to the current waves of instability and fear so many of us are experiencing.

Discover how to identify the angels living amongst us and why we all have light-bodies. You will have the opportunity to find the ultimate God within you and discover why a God seen as separate from yourself keeps you from being in your Divine Power and happiness. In addition, you can find out how to heal yourself at a moment's notice. Read all about the 'New Medicine' and the destiny of the old medicine, the old economy, the old religion, and the old world.

It's Time to Come Alive!
Start Using the Amazing Healing Powers of Your Body, Mind, and Spirit Today!

In this book, the author brings to light man's deep inner need for spiritual wisdom in life and helps the reader develop a new sense of reality that is based on love, power, and compassion. He describes our relationship with the natural world in detail and discusses how we can harness its tremendous powers for our personal benefit and that of humanity. *It's Time to Come Alive* challenges some of our most commonly held beliefs and offers a way out of the emotional restrictions and physical limitations we have created in our lives.

Topics include: What shapes our destiny; using the power of intention; secrets of defying the aging process; doubting – the cause of failure; opening the heart; material wealth and spiritual wealth; fatigue – the major cause of stress; methods of emotional transformation; techniques of primordial healing; how to increase the health of the five senses; developing spiritual wisdom; the major causes of today's earth changes; entry into the new world; twelve gateways to heaven on earth; and many more.

Feel Great, Lose Weight
Stop Dieting and Start Living

No rigorous workouts. No surgery. In this book, celebrated author Andreas Moritz suggests a gentle – and permanent – route to losing weight. In this ground-breaking book, he says that once we stop blaming our genes and take control of our own life, weight-loss is a natural consequence.

"You need to make that critical mental shift. You need to experience the willingness to shed your physical and emotional baggage, not by counting calories but by embracing your mind, body and spirit. Once you start looking at yourself differently, 80 percent of the work is done."

In Feel Great, Lose Weight, Andreas Moritz tells us why conventional weight-loss programs don't work and how weight-loss 'experts' make sure we keep going back. He also tells us why food manufacturers, pharmaceutical companies and health regulators conspire to keep America toxically overweight.

But we can refuse to buy into the Big Fat Lie. Choosing the mind-body approach triggers powerful biochemical changes that set us on a safe and irreversible path to losing weight, without resorting to crash diets, heavy workouts or dangerous surgical procedures.

Simple Steps to Total Health!
Andreas Moritz with co-author John Hornecker

By nature, your physical body is designed to be healthy and vital throughout life. Unhealthy eating habits and lifestyle choices, however, lead to numerous health conditions that prevent you from enjoying life to the fullest. In *Simple Steps to Total Health*, the authors bring to light the most common cause of disease, which is the buildup of toxins and residues from improperly digested foods that inhibit various organs and systems from performing their normal functions. This guidebook for total health provides you with simple but highly effective approaches for internal cleansing, hydration, nutrition, and living habits.

The book's three parts cover the essentials of total health - Good Internal Hygiene, Healthy Nutrition, and Balanced Lifestyle. Learn about the most common disease-causing foods, dietary habits and influences responsible for the occurrence of chronic illnesses, including those affecting the blood vessels, heart, liver, intestinal organs, lungs, kidneys, joints, bones, nervous system, and sense organs.

To be able to live a healthy life, you must align your internal biological rhythms with the larger rhythms of nature. Find out more about this and many other important topics in *Simple Steps to Total Health*. This is a 'must-have' book for anyone who is interested in using a natural, drug-free approach to restore total health.

Heart Disease No More!
Make Peace with Your Heart and Heal Yourself
(Excerpted from Timeless Secrets of
Health and Rejuvenation)

Less than a hundred years ago, heart disease was an extremely rare illness. Today it kills more people in the developed world than all other causes of death combined. Despite the vast quantity of financial resources spent on finding a cure for heart disease, the current medical approaches remain mainly symptom-oriented and do not address the underlying causes.

Even worse, overwhelming evidence shows that the treatment of heart disease or its presumed precursors, such as high blood pressure, hardening of the arteries, and high cholesterol, not only prevents a real cure, but also can easily lead to chronic heart failure. The patient's heart may still beat, but not strongly enough for him to feel vital and alive.

Without removing the underlying causes of heart disease and its precursors, the average person has little, if any, protection against it. Heart attacks can strike whether you have undergone a coronary bypass or have had stents placed inside your arteries. According to research, these procedures fail to prevent heart attacks and do nothing to reduce mortality rates.

Heart Disease No More, excerpted from the author's bestselling book, Timeless Secrets of Health and Rejuvenation, puts the responsibility for healing where it belongs, on the heart, mind, and body of each individual. It provides the reader with practical insights about the development and causes of heart disease. Even better, it explains simple steps you can take to prevent and reverse heart disease for good, regardless of a possible genetic predisposition.

Diabetes - No More!
Discover and Heal Its True Causes
(Excerpted from Timeless Secrets of Health and Rejuvenation)

According to this bestselling author, diabetes is not a disease; in the vast majority of cases, it is a complex mechanism of protection or survival that the body chooses to avoid the possibly fatal consequences of an unhealthful diet and lifestyle.

Despite the body's ceaseless self-preservation efforts (which we call diseases), millions of people suffer or die unnecessarily from these consequences. The imbalanced blood sugar level in diabetes is but a symptom of illness, not the illness itself. By developing diabetes, the body is neither doing something wrong, nor is it trying to commit suicide. The current diabetes epidemic is man-made, or rather, factory-made, and, therefore, can be halted and reversed through simple but effective changes in diet and lifestyle. *Diabetes – No More* provides you with essential information on the various causes of diabetes and how anyone can avoid them.

To stop the diabetes epidemic you need to create the right circumstances that allow your body to heal. Just as there is a mechanism to become diabetic, there is also a mechanism to reverse it. Find out how!

This book was excerpted from the bestselling book, *Timeless Secrets of Health and Rejuvenation.*

Ending The AIDS Myth
It's Time to Heal the TRUE Causes!
(Excerpted from Timeless Secrets of Health and Rejuvenation)

Contrary to common belief, no scientific evidence exists to this day to prove that AIDS is a contagious disease. The current AIDS theory falls short in predicting the kind of AIDS disease an infected person may be manifesting, and no accurate system is in place to determine how long it will take for the disease to develop. In addition, the current HIV/AIDS theory contains no reliable information that can help identify those who are at risk for developing AIDS.

On the other hand, published research actually proves that HIV only spreads through heterosexually in extremely rare cases and cannot be responsible for an epidemic that involves millions of AIDS victims around the world. Furthermore, it is an established fact that the retrovirus HIV, which is composed of human gene fragments, is incapable of destroying human cells. However, cell destruction is the main characteristic of every AIDS disease.

Even the principal discoverer of HIV, Luc Montagnier, no longer believes that HIV is solely responsible for causing AIDS. In fact, he showed that HIV alone could not cause AIDS. Increasing evidence indicates that AIDS may be a toxicity syndrome or metabolic disorder that is caused by immunity risk factors, including heroin, sex-enhancement drugs, antibiotics, commonly prescribed AIDS drugs, rectal intercourse, starvation, malnutrition, and dehydration

Dozens of prominent scientists working at the forefront of AIDS research now openly question the virus hypothesis of AIDS. Find out why! Ending the AIDS Myth also shows you what really causes the shutdown of the immune system and what you can do to avoid this.

267

Heal Yourself with Sunlight
Use Its Secret Medicinal Powers to Help Cure Cancer,
Heart Disease, Hypertension, Diabetes Arthritis,
Infectious Diseases, and much more.

This book by Andreas Moritz provides scientific evidence that sunlight is essential for good health, and that a lack of sun exposure can be held responsible for many of today's diseases.

On the other hand, most people now believe that the sun is the main culprit for causing skin cancer, certain cataracts leading to blindness, and aging. Only those who take the risk of exposing themselves to the sunlight, find that the sun makes them feel and look better, provided they don't use sunscreens or burn their skin. The UV-rays in sunlight actually stimulate the thyroid gland to increase hormone production, which in turn increases the body's basal metabolic rate. This assists both in weight loss and improved muscle development.

It has been known for several decades that those living mostly in the outdoors, at high altitudes, or near the equator, have the lowest incidence of skin cancers. In addition, studies revealed that exposing patients to controlled amounts of sunlight dramatically lowered elevated blood pressure (up to 40 mm Hg drop), decreased cholesterol in the blood stream, lowered abnormally high blood sugars among diabetics, and increased the number of white blood cells which we need to help resist disease. Patients suffering from gout, rheumatoid arthritis, colitis, arteriosclerosis, anemia, cystitis, eczema, acne, psoriasis, herpes, lupus, sciatica, kidney problems, asthma, as well as burns, have all shown to receive great benefit from the healing rays of the sun.

Hear the Whispers, Live Your Dream
A Fanfare of Inspiration

Listening to the whispers of your heart will set you free. The beauty and bliss of your knowingness and love center are what we are here to capture, take in and swim with. You are like a dolphin sailing in a sea of joy. Allow yourself to open to the wondrous fullness of your selfhood, without reservation and without judgment.

Judgment stands in the way, like a boulder trespassing on your journey to the higher reaches of your destiny. Push these boulders aside and feel the joy of your inner truth sprout forth. Do not allow another's thoughts or directions for you to supersede your inner knowingness, for you relinquish being the full, radiant star that you are.

It is with an open heart, a receptive mind, and a reaching for the stars of wisdom that lie within you, that you reap the bountiful goodness of mother Earth and the universal I AM. For you are a benevolent being of light and there is no course that can truly stop you, except your own thoughts, or allowing another's beliefs to override your own.

May these aphorisms of love, joy and wisdom inspire you to be the wondrous being that you were born to be!

All books are available in paperback and as electronic books through the Ener-Chi Wellness Center

Website: http://www.ener-chi.com
Email: support@ener-chi.com

Toll free 1(866) 258-4006 (USA)
Local: 1(709) 570-7401 (Canada)

Index

274

275

Pastuer, Louis, xi, 3-4
PEDIATRICS, 12
PedvaxHIB vaccine recall, 57
Perry, Rick, 65
Pertussis vaccine
adverse events pertaining to, 46
effectiveness of, 136
encephalitis risk with, 53
PFNYC. *See* Partnership for New York City
Pharma-media-vaccine-dollars connection, 174-175
Placebo effect, 219, 220
Placebo fraud
impact on medical treatment, 223-224
pharmaceutical drugs comparison with placebo pills, 221, 222
Placebos
composition influence on trial outcomes, 221
drug makers discretion in selecting, 222
inert, problems in getting, 222
lactose in AIDS drugs testing, 224
used in heart studies, 222
Plasma cells and healing process, 13
Pneumonia, 61
causes of, 194-195
treatment with antibiotics, 195
Polio, overhauling definition of, 36-37
Polio vaccination
adverse events linked with, 68-69
number of polio cases following, 34
Polio vaccine
and acanthamoeba, link between, 58
contamination with SV40 virus, 29-30, 162
immune reaction to, 31
neurological 'syndromes' due to, 120
Polysorbate 80, side effects of, 25
Porcine circovirus PCV1, 134
Preservatives
neurological damage by, 146-147
Prevnar pneumococcal 7-valent Conjugate vaccine recall, 57
Probodies, 10
Professional misconduct, 77-79
Psychological traumas, classification of, 213
Public ignorance and immunization programs, 44-45
Quackery, 85
Reassortment process, 162, 176
Re-diagnosis of diseases, 37-39

Red measles vaccine, 37
Residual agents, 23
Retrovirus, 73
Rheumatoid arthritis, 115-116
Rho-Gam, 142
Rotarix
contamination with pig virus, 134
FDA study on, 133
Routes of entry
attenuated virus of vaccines, 51
body response to, 61
pathogens, 51
Rubella virus, growth of, 23
Sabin, Albert, 120, 205
Salk, Jonas, 1, 30
Sanofi Pasteur, vaccine recall by, 56
SBS. *See* Shaken Baby Syndrome
Scheibner, Viera, 116
Science (journal), 1
Scientific misconduct surveys, 79-80
Scientific research, flaws in, 86-88
Seasonal flu. *See* Flu
Self-healing, 219
Self-immunization practices, 13-14
Shaken Baby Syndrome, 54
Shingles
clinical features, 48
risk following chickenpox vaccination, 47
Shingles vaccine, 49
SIDS. *See* Sudden Infant Death Syndrome
Simian Vacuolating Virus 40 (SV40), polio vaccine contamination with, 29-30, 54
Smallpox, re-diagnosis of, 39
Smallpox vaccine
components of, 32
smallpox outbreak following, 31-32
Snake venom
acquisition of human immunity against, 13
constituents of, 14
immune reaction to exposure to, 14
Spanish avian flu outbreak, 195
Special Virus Cancer Program, 72
Spontaneous regression, 214-215
Squalene
autoimmune disorders caused by, 186-187
autoimmune response triggered by, 63-64
characteristics of, 185
use in vaccines, 186-187
Stabilizing agents, 53
concerns regarding, 23
functions of, 23

276

9 780984 595426